"I have a chronic illness that was misdiagnosed for decades. Countless doctor visits and a fleet of alternative remedies not only brought no real relief but added to the shame, pain, confusion, isolation, and sense of failure I often felt during those years. What I needed most was a companion like Liuan Huska—someone who had not only walked a similar difficult journey but had done the emotional, theological, and medical work that could bring wisdom and insight to the questions that arise around chronic illness. *Hurting Yet Whole* is a book brimming with honesty about the nature of what it is to be an embodied human being made in the image of God. There are no quick fixes or simple formulas in this beautiful book, but there is something of much greater value in its pages for patients, caregivers, pastors, and anyone who loves someone facing an ongoing illness: compassion."

Michelle Van Loon, author of *Becoming Sage: Cultivating Maturity, Purpose, and Spirituality in Midlife*

"We have another theologian on our hands! Here you have a wise, studied, and informative look at living as an embodied human being. While reflecting on her own story, Liuan Huska thinks carefully and writes well about the meaning of wholeness given our illnesses or chronic illnesses. What's more, she highlights a looming problem: our penchant for swimming in a sea of modern-day Gnosticism (among other things). This book is powerful because it is a lived theology, a practical theology of the body in narrative form, not detached speculation. Incarnational. May we sit at her feet and learn."

Marlena Graves, author of *The Way Up Is Down: Finding Yourself by Forgetting Yourself* and *A Beautiful Disaster*

"*Hurting Yet Whole* is a welcome addition to the literature about living with chronic illness. Liuan Huska weaves her personal experience with theological insight in an accessible and compelling way. This would be a deeply helpful resource for people just beginning to grapple with the reality of chronic illness in their own lives, and anyone desiring to respond to the limits, pains, and contingencies of their own physical body with less enmity and more tenderness."

Bethany McKinney Fox, director of student success and adjunct professor of Christian ethics at Fuller Theological Seminary, author of *Disability and the Way of Jesus*

"*Hurting Yet Whole* speaks to an issue every Christian—every person— faces: How do we live well in bodies that don't always work 'right'? Every human on the planet has, or will, experience the 'malfunctioning' of our own bodies. But is this only about loss? Can we only think of this in terms of what is wrong? How have those who have gone before us and members of diverse cultures thought about and experienced these same phenomena? In the vein of Malcolm Gladwell or Andy Crouch, Liuan Huska has made accessible sophisticated research from areas such as anthropology, biology, psychology, and theology, together with narratives of her own and others, to offer this gift of a book. If you have a body or know someone who does, this book is for you."

Brian M. Howell, professor of anthropology at Wheaton College

"There's a lot of bad theology on suffering to suffer through. Liuan Huska's *Hurting Yet Whole* does the hard work of sifting through the mire and offering us a finer answer to the eternal question, How do I live in my body now?"

Erin S. Lane, author of *Lessons in Belonging from a Church-Going Commitment Phobe*

"Liuan Huska has woven her own story of chronic pain together with theological critique and insight in a way that is both easily accessible and deeply thoughtful. This book is not just a hopeful and honest guide for people suffering from physical ailments. It is also a companion into the pain of a fragmented and disconnected world that longs to be made whole. *Hurting Yet Whole* invites all of us to understand pain differently than our culture—and the church—has taught us, so that we can find a different type of healing and wholeness."

Amy Julia Becker, author of *White Picket Fences: Turning toward Love in a World Divided by Privilege*

"Of all people, Christians should have an understanding and appreciation of the human bodies God created that bear his image. Yet, too often, Christians neglect the role our bodies play in the life of our souls on earth and in eternity. I'm so thankful for the way Liuan Huska tenderly and humanely stitches these two parts of our humanity back together in this wise, lovely book."

Karen Swallow Prior, author of *On Reading Well* and *Fierce Convictions*

LIUAN HUSKA

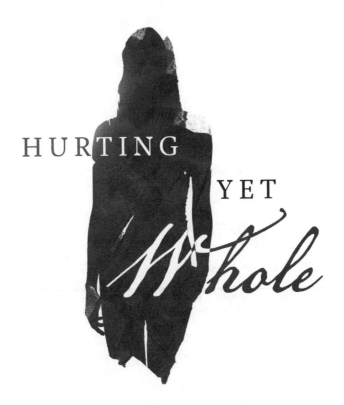

HURTING
YET
Whole

RECONCILING BODY AND SPIRIT
IN CHRONIC PAIN AND ILLNESS

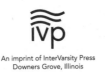

An imprint of InterVarsity Press
Downers Grove, Illinois

InterVarsity Press
P.O. Box 1400, Downers Grove, IL 60515-1426
ivpress.com
email@ivpress.com

InterVarsity Press® is the book-publishing division of InterVarsity Christian Fellowship/USA®, a movement of students and faculty active on campus at hundreds of universities, colleges, and schools of nursing in the United States of America, and a member movement of the International Fellowship of Evangelical Students. For information about local and regional activities, visit intervarsity.org.

Scripture quotations, unless otherwise noted, are from the New Revised Standard Version Bible, copyright © 1989 National Council of the Churches of Christ in the United States of America. Used by permission. All rights reserved worldwide.

While any stories in this book are true, some names and identifying information may have been changed to protect the privacy of individuals.

Cover design and image composite: David Fassett
Interior design: Daniel van Loon
Image: grungy black border: © blackred / iStock / Getty Images

ISBN 978-0-8308-4807-2 (print)
ISBN 978-0-8308-4808-9 (digital)

Printed in the United States of America ♾

Library of Congress Cataloging-in-Publication Data
A catalog record for this book is available from the Library of Congress.

P	21	20	19	18	17	16	15	14	13	12	11	10	9	8	7	6	5	4	3	2	1
Y	37	36	35	34	33	32	31	30	29	28	27	26	25	24	23	22	21	20

TO MY BOYS

May you each be part of the healing of this world.

CONTENTS

1

A JOURNEY BEGINS

We come into this world blissfully unaware of these fragile, beautiful things we call our bodies. In our mother's womb, we bathe in continuous warmth and nourishment, changing shadows and muffled voices, not knowing where our mothers end and where we begin. We are one. We are whole.

Out in the bright, chilly world, most of us pass through childhood in a similar ignorance of unmediated bodily immediacy.[1] We reach out to touch, smell, and taste all the blankets, fingers, dirt clods, oranges, chair legs, and windblown leaves we encounter. Our bodies move and grow, and sometimes get hurt and heal, without our thinking much about it.

Many of us also enter adulthood thinking very little about our bodies. They are just . . . there. They may alert us of their presence if we stub our toe on the bed frame in a nighttime bathroom expedition or when the powdery yellow coat of spring pollen irritates our sinuses. Mainly, though, bodies are the taken-for-granted backdrop to all we do in life. Our feet walk us through the grocery store, our fingers and eyes facilitate our internet browsing, our noses and skin take in the presence of our loved ones. But we don't notice our bodies in these moments. They just do what they're supposed to do. And we go on living.

Then there comes a time when our bodies stop doing what they're supposed to. They leap from their benign presence in the background and scream for attention. We can't help but notice. We ache. We double over. We can't walk, can't think, can't breathe. Something isn't right. Our bodies fall apart.

For many, this awareness comes with aging. My mother often groans, "I feel like I am getting old." Bodily deterioration—rickety joints, sagging skin, the slowing march of internal organs—is a normal, decades-long part of the business of living that leads to dying that leads to death—the complete halt of bodily function.

For a growing number of us, though, our bodies malfunction long before normal aging sets in. Something goes wrong and refuses to be fixed by one or two visits to the doctor and time. Some of us have joints that start to swell and ache as teenagers. Others have jackhammer headaches that debilitate us for days. Yet others live with fatigue that makes the word *tired* seem like child's play.

For me, it was a niggling pain in my left ankle that spread to my foot, knee, back, and neck. After months of frustrating doctor's visits, varying diagnoses, and ineffective treatments, I just started calling it "chronic pain." Whatever name we end up giving our ailments, whatever treatments we endure, we share the feeling of a sudden disconnect with our bodies. It's not just that we are getting old. "From the moment we are born, we begin to die," the saying goes. When we have a chronic illness, our bodies do not recover the way they should from an injury or change in the internal ecosystem. We don't bounce back. We languish. Our bodies, once friends that came along for the ride, become our betrayers—all-consuming burdens of pain and frustration that thwart our goals and our chance to live a "normal" life.

FALLING APART

Before pain, I was invincible. The world was my oyster. I was twenty-two, just out of college, and plotting my globetrotting, book-writing path through God's green earth. When the pain first started, I didn't give it much thought. It was some minor sprain, probably, that would go away with time. When weeks turned to months and I was still not able to walk more than a few blocks, the pain began taking up more real estate in my mind. *What is going on? Why isn't it getting better?*

I began to mistrust my body, which had once served me so well. I distanced myself. In my heart and mind, I stepped out of my body and away from the pain, vulnerability, and limits it represented. I told myself I shouldn't be having such a disproportionate level of fear and anxiety over a minor injury. After all, it was just my body that was hurt. I—that is, my personhood, my locus of self, the consciousness that experiences the world—was still okay. Right?

Over and over, I found this wasn't the case. Pain covered my whole self and my experiences like a veil. Life, even the most profound, celebratory moments (or perhaps especially those), took on a purplish, grayish tint. About a year into the pain, for example, on a lovely summer evening, my husband and I attended our friends' wedding reception in their apartment complex courtyard. I put on an airy dress and tennis shoes, determined to enjoy myself and ignore the spasms and pinpricks in my back and ankle. Neighborhood refugee children from Sudan and Burma shrieked and threaded through the tables while we devoured homemade tacos and salsa. When the music started, people of so many skin hues and accents streamed onto the patch of grass under strings of lights hung across the balconies. It was a beautiful picture of togetherness and harmony.

I had to join in. Dragging my husband, Matt, into the edge of the moving mass, I let the rhythm carry me. As I moved, though, the static noise of pain in my body rose over the other sensations—the freewheeling elation of dancing, children's yells, Shakira's voice through the speakers. For a brief moment, I had emerged from the cave of pain to join the world of the living. And then, so quickly, my body pulled me back into that cave. The angry, twitching knots in my muscles and joints took over my senses like a waterfall pounding down, drowning out sight and sound, veiling the outside world. The world of a person in pain, essayist Elaine Scarry writes, shrinks to the confines of her body.[2]

I retreated to my seat, trying to convince myself that I could enjoy this party just as well without dancing, but something in my bones told otherwise. I was made to dance, made to express joy through movement. If I couldn't find a way to be fully present in my body, then something was missing. Some part of my life was inaccessible. This sense of "missing-ness" caused more pain than the physical pain itself.

PAIN AND ITS COHORTS

The connection between my body and my being, which I had taken for granted growing up, was fraying. The pain forced me to step back and see my body in a strange new light. What mysterious, malignant forces were working within it to cause me such suffering? How could I have walked about so blithely when at any moment cancer could strike, some environmental toxin could wreak havoc in my cells, or I could fall and break a bone and never recover due to some weird disease I might have? I could no longer trust my body. It was no longer good. I couldn't accept that my body was part of me, if it was this sack of disorder. It was Other. Or, if I really was my body and we were inseparable, did that mean I was broken and decaying at my core?

As I wailed over my uncooperative body, the depression, fear and anxiety began swallowing me whole. Every odd symptom fed hypochondria and dismay. The life I had once envisioned no longer fit my current reality. Instead of plotting the realization of my pet projects, my thoughts drifted toward tragedy.

One Thursday, in the middle of my job at the county courthouse, an email slipped into my inbox from the church office. I read and reread it, not comprehending. "Yesterday around 9:10 p.m. Jonan Eilam Pelletier was birthed to parents Jeff and Kimberly. He had passed away some time on Monday." Was birthed. Had passed away. How could someone be birthed when he had already passed away? It took me a while to realize Jonan Eilam had died in the womb.

I closed out the email and continued pecking at my keyboard, entering the names and addresses of the day's delinquents for my boss to send to lawyers, who would then mail these petty criminals to offer their services. But Jonan Eilam stayed with me long after I shut the laptop, drove home, and collapsed on the futon, my routine in those days. I felt a strange communion with him, as if he were a fellow soldier who had fallen. It seemed morbid, but I was drawn to something about Jonan Eilam's short life and much-too-early death. I wanted to turn away, because I felt like an intruder peering in on a neighbor family's private grief. But I couldn't stop thinking about him.

Maybe this was why: knowing that others also deal with sudden loss made my own losses more bearable. I wasn't the only one. Life *was* crazy, just like it seemed. Other people were also asking *why*. Why do some bodies work and others fall apart? Why did Jonan Eilam die before birth while others live past one hundred? Why did my ankle start hurting out of nowhere while others put their joints through marathons and mountain climbs, coming out the other end just fine?

Perhaps, I thought, I was a bit like Jonan Eilam. My body and heart were also fragile and weak, maybe not strong enough for the crushing weight of living. Sometimes I longed to slip with him into a place where it was easier to breathe, where gravity didn't pull us down. That night, I penned in my journal, "Life is too much sometimes, for Jonan Eilam and me."

These kinds of thoughts pulled me apart from others in terrifying ways. The people closest to me looked on with concern but couldn't get down to those darkest places, where rational thought and hope slipped away. They couldn't jump out of their skin and into mine. And, as I discovered with my husband, they were humans with their own needs, limited in their ability to be there for me at those most inconvenient times when panic attacked.

It usually happened deep into the night, after I'd flopped around for hours like a dying fish trying to get comfortable, when I had nothing to distract me from the low whine of throbbing joints and fearful thoughts. One of those nights, not long after the apartment complex wedding, the thoughts came swarming, biting, pegging themselves onto my chest in droves so I could hardly breathe. *What if it's like this for the rest of my life? Or what if the pain just gets worse and worse and I end up confined to bed? How can it have only been two years since that beautiful, rainbow-tinted day when we got married? We've spent half of our marriage with me in pain, complaining. What a drag for Matt. Now that I have nothing to look forward to in life, what am I even living for? How can I bear the rest of my life if it's like this?*

I tried repeating the Jesus Prayer. "Lord Jesus Christ, Son of God, have mercy on me, a sinner." Over and over and over. Still, the internal noise of anxiety rose, and I thought my chest might explode. I needed to do something, anything.

I turned to shake Matt. He groaned in an irritated sleep-drawl, "Whaaaat?"

"I can't sleep," I whispered timidly.

This was the umpteenth time I had woken him in the middle of the night to replay my fears and cry into his chest. I waited for him to turn and ask me what was wrong this time. To re-assure me that I was going to be okay. Instead, he muttered, "I need to sleep, Liuan! Can't it wait till morning?" and rolled over with his back to me.

If I had been hanging on by a thread, that thread snapped. Though my rational mind told me that it *could* wait, that nothing would change by telling Matt the same things I'd already told him a hundred times before, my heart was like a wild animal, trapped and getting more frenzied by the second. I crawled out of bed into the shadowy living room and stared. Then, sprawling on the floor in my blue and white checkered nightgown, I grabbed the nearest object, a jacket, and slammed it into the floor. I did this again and again, listening to the zipper and cloth slap against the wood and bounce off, working myself into a fever. I pounded my fists into the floor and gave voice to my demons. The sounds were guttural, choked, and shocking. I was trapped in the cage of my own body. I couldn't even go outside to run it out. I was alone, and I couldn't leave.

At some point, Matt did get up. I guess I forced him to, with my foaming-at-the-mouth demonstration. He wrapped his arms around me. His tight grip and his chest—warm and solid—against my back gave me a reference point outside of my own unreliable skin and bones. I let the fury and fear tumbling inside me drain into another body. The buzzing swarm on my chest lifted, for a moment. I somehow managed to go back to bed and face another day.

DARK NIGHT OF THE SOUL

I struggled to patch my faith onto the growing hole of despair in my core. There were no easy answers. I wanted to be healed. I wanted to be whole. Wholeness is a unity of parts, a fitting together of pieces into a seamless, coherent entity. I was anything but whole. I was falling apart on so many levels.

Though I could draw from a rich legacy of theodicy, people defending the goodness of God against the reality of evil, words fall short in the face of human suffering. I started asking questions that not many people I knew cared to answer. Questions like, *if the healing work of Jesus applies to the whole of us, including our bodies, what does that mean when you're always hurting? Can my fragile, suffering body offer anything to my understanding of a meaningful life, or must 1 ignore it in order to go on?*

Traditional Christian views that tell us we are more than our bodies only helped so much. Paul says in 2 Corinthians 4:16, "Even though our outer nature is wasting away, our inner nature is being renewed day by day." I have always understood this verse to be Paul's way of dealing with the reality of our fragile, broken bodies. He is saying, "Okay, your bones may be losing density, your hair falling out, and your blood vessels clogging, but your soul is alive and well." Some strands of Christianity take this even further, teaching that our body doesn't matter; all that matters is our eternal soul. Wholeness is only important in that we are spiritually whole, in right relationship with God and others. Body and soul live in separate realms and don't mix. We go to the doctor to deal with our bodies, and to church to deal with our souls.

I internalized versions of these messages, some that others told me and some that I told myself: "Liuan, you have to be able to tell God, 'I will love and serve you with one good foot or two.'" "You can still be part of God's kingdom, regardless of what's going on in your body." "Look at all that you still have—your family, a loving husband, friends, a job, graduate school. Don't focus so much on your body. Just trust God. It will get better." These messages were encouraging to some extent, lifting my gaze off my health woes and onto a larger reality. In other ways, they deepened the disconnect I felt with my own body and my disillusionment with the church.

I couldn't find many people concerned with the nagging questions I had about how to reconnect my poor aching body with my poor aching soul. Rather, my suffering was often spiritualized by others. Once, I went up to a prayer minister at a church I was visiting. After listening attentively to my story, the woman asked, "Are you harboring any unforgiveness in your heart?" People in church tried to answer the unanswerable whys, claiming my pain was punishment, a test of character, or intended by God to accomplish some other end. But none of their answers addressed the question I was asking: How do I live in my body now? The gulf continued to widen between me and the body of Christ. Another instance of falling apart.

Finally, there was my relationship with God. As my depression and pain worsened and prayers for healing remained unanswered, my once vibrant prayer life, where I heard and saw tangible evidence of God's care for me, seemed to diminish to me moaning at the wall in my room. God appeared to have gone on vacation to Fiji.

I felt plunged into what St. John of the Cross described as the "dark night of the soul." It can be a rich place of deepening faith and spiritual maturity. The pilgrim gropes toward God not based on sight, but on faith. Going through it, though, is terrifying. That unshakable conviction I had in the past that all would be well in the end faltered. I questioned all I knew about God and how he worked. If God was good, and what was going on in my life was somehow part of his good purposes, then I wasn't so sure I wanted the "good" he had to offer. I was afraid to draw near to God, who was no longer the comforting, ever-present God I had known. I was afraid that maybe, if I pushed deeper, God would turn out to be shadows in the fog, a figment of my own wishful thinking. So I kept my distance from God. I stayed apart.

BECOMING WHOLE

It has been ten years now since the pain first started. Since then I have finished a master's degree, started freelance writing, and become a mother to three little boys. I still have pain, but it's not nearly as much of a presence as it used to be. It comes and goes, though it never fully leaves. Certain positions, like sleeping frequently on my left side, and certain activities, like walking in flat shoes without support, bring it all back. When I get too physically ambitious, the pain is like an old friend who calls to say, "I know where you come from—dust and ashes. Ha! You can't fool me!"

I've learned to accept what my body is. Sometimes, even, like when I pushed a ten-and-a-half-pound firstborn out, I marvel at it.

I have wondered in these years if the ways we understand healing might not have contributed to my falling apart. What *is* healing, when one has a chronic illness? Can a person still be whole (not just spiritually whole, but *wholly* whole) when her body is not functioning properly and she is suffering? I believe so, though it takes some unlearning of what we have assumed the good, successful life to be.

I'd like to sketch a different vision of healing, one seared by unrelenting brokenness, pain, and disease. To heal, as I understand it, is to become whole.

The educator Parker Palmer writes, "Wholeness doesn't mean perfection: It means embracing brokenness as an integral part of life." When Palmer speaks of wholeness, he doesn't mean a perfectly functioning body, or even a worldview where all the pieces fit together. What he has in mind is closer to the idea of *integrity*. He uses Douglas Wood's meditation on a jack pine to illustrate:

> Jack pines . . . are not lumber trees [and they] won't win many beauty contests either. But to me this valiant old tree, solitary on its own rocky point, is as beautiful as a living thing can be. . . . In the calligraphy of its shape against the sky is written strength of character and perseverance, survival of wind, drought, cold, heat, disease. . . . In its silence it speaks of . . . wholeness . . . an integrity that comes from being what you are.[3]

Being who you are. For many, chronic illness pulls the rug out from under our old identities, interests, and life pursuits. We no longer know who we are, or who God is. We must find a new way to be.

It is tempting to wish to go back to a previous state, that "normal" life we had when good health was assumed, our bodies were reliable, and God could be found. Too many of us cling to this flimsy ideal when we desperately seek treatment and healing. But as my disillusionment with God and the church deepened and I realized that pain was unavoidable, I knew I couldn't go back to the old normal. I knew too much darkness, too much loss, that I couldn't unknow. Theologian Marva Dawn calls this a loss of innocence, a loss of certainty.[4]

It's hard to imagine any other way to be whole than feeling sure of a good life ahead, with health, career success, family, financial stability—all those things people say are your birthright (if you are a middle-class white American, that is). As I have let go of these things as givens and stared at the broken pieces straight on, however, I have sensed that there *has* to be another way to be whole.

BECOMING FULLY HUMAN

If wholeness, as Parker Palmer hints at, is this ability to *be who you are*, then I want to be who I am now fully. I want to integrate these experiences of suffering and brokenness into my being—how I see the world and God and myself in it. I want to take my pain, this truth that I now know in my tendons and ligaments, and hold it up against the gospel of Jesus Christ—his incarnation, death, resurrection, and promise of second coming. Will there be resonance, connection, unity . . . wholeness? Will the gospel illuminate my experiences? Will my experiences illuminate the gospel?

In fact, the Christian story has a lot to say to our pain. While some may think of faith as victory over pain and suffering (which it is ultimately), what we see in Jesus' life is not an escape from the everyday drag of having a body, but an embrace. Including all the discomforts, inconveniences, and embarrassments that come with it. *God became a human body.* What's more—*God still is a human body now in the resurrected Christ.*

I will explore this truth from the perspective of chronic illness. Healing is not an escape from the limits, vulnerabilities, and suffering of the body, but rather, it is becoming whole—becoming *who we are.* We are souls in bodies, but we are also bodies with souls. We will never *not* be bodies, even though implicit messages we have heard in the church may have misled us to believe we will one day shrug off all physical encumbrances. The new creation, theologian N. T. Wright declares, will be "a new kind of physicality, which will not need to decay and die . . . *more* physical, more solid, more utterly real."[5]

To heal, to become whole, we must embrace the truth of who we are—a triune personhood of body, mind, and soul—in light of who our triune God is. We must learn to be fully human, not *super*human, by living within our embodied limits, not transcending them. We must make peace with our tenuous existence, susceptible at any moment to devastating illnesses and even death. We must realize that our vulnerability is what opens us to relying on others, and, through these relationships, becoming whole.

Chronic illness, though a tragedy, forces us to pay attention to our bodies. Due to our longer life spans as well as other factors, a growing number of people have chronic illnesses—conditions that go on indeterminately and don't respond quickly to treatment.[6] Some of these illnesses, like heart disease and diabetes, are widely recognized and can be managed by standard treatments (though they are still difficult to bear). Others are "invisible illnesses" that don't manifest in measurable, obvious ways (fibromyalgia, chronic fatigue, and lupus are examples). These bring added suffering due to the lack of recognition and social support. This book is for all who struggle to make sense of how the God of the gospel meets us in our broken bodies, especially those who have felt unheard and unsupported.

A WAY FORWARD

In the coming chapters, I will deconstruct and reconstruct our understanding of wholeness. I will also share my own story and bring in the voices of others who have graciously entrusted their stories to me. Over coffee, phone, video chat, and email, these people have let me interview them, allowing me into those hurting, wondering places where God and illness do not make sense. Their stories, which are interspersed with my own, do not have a neat bow tied at the end. They are stories of people wrestling, questioning, staggering, sometimes making peace, sometimes not. These are the stories I wish I had heard in the valleys of pain. They ring true and speak to our resilience. If we can press into them, and not shy away from the shadowy spots where meaning evaporates and only groans remain, maybe we will find, in the darkest pits, the God who descended even deeper, who shows us a way through to new life.

Though I use chronic illness as a lens, my questions are not unique to that experience. The aging and disabled also know bodily limits and vulnerability well. Admittedly, what I describe here is the experience of being thrust into pain or illness in the middle of life, often abruptly. This is different (though not necessarily harder or easier) than being born with a disability or illness and learning early on how to accept these givens and integrate body and identity. For example, many in the deaf community don't see their deafness as *lack of* hearing, but as a culture with its own language and meanings. Those in the disability community have paved the way for the rest of us to reimagine our identities and bodies against the grain of "normal" functioning.[7]

Aging, on the other hand, is an expected life stage, though this doesn't make the loss of physical capacities any more bearable. Mental illness, too, brings to the surface the depths of our human condition—our darkness, our unchecked impulses, our lack of control over our external and even internal states of being.[8] Many of these categories overlap, and often one leads to another. Illness, for instance, might lead to a permanent disability, or chronic pain might lead to depression and anxiety (as it did in my case), which are forms of mental illness. And all of us, at one point or another, will have some of these experiences. Though we often see our health and able-bodied capacities as the default, it would be more accurate to see them as the extreme end of a spectrum, with most of us falling somewhere in the middle and moving back and forth throughout our lives.

Because my questions are not unique to chronic illness, I hope my reflections will benefit not only those with chronic illness, but all of us who follow our enfleshed Lord. We are all members of him, and of one another. We have, sadly, often dismissed experiences of chronic illness because we prefer tidy stories of immediate healing. We'd rather cling to our ten-step formulas and the misguided hope that if we follow the rules and do the right things, we will avoid major suffering. If we take chronic illness seriously, we must question these assumptions. We must face pain and suffering as unavoidable realities of life and find ways to integrate these experiences into our life vision. We must open ourselves to lament, paradox, and mystery. In doing so, we will find ourselves joined to each other in a unity deeper than our aching bones, joined to God who binds all our wounds and makes something more, something beautiful, out of it all.

May we journey closer to this kind of wholeness. May those with chronic illness and pain embrace their hurting yet still-so-wonderful bodies. May the church embrace her broken yet still-so-necessary members. May we heal from ways of thinking that dishonor our bodies and deepen the rifts between our bodies, minds, and spirits.

Lord Jesus Christ, have mercy upon us. Lord Jesus Christ, make us whole.

PART ONE

Falling

APART

2

SPLIT AT THE CORE

I studied at a Christian liberal arts college where chapel attendance was required three times a week and Communion was offered once a month. During one evening Communion service, I saw something unusual. As students went up to receive the elements and the chapel band played, a few women left their seats and headed to the side aisles next to the stage. Then they started sashaying, twirling, leaping, and raising their arms and legs in graceful and expressive movements. They were dancing at Communion.

As a dancer myself, I appreciated their outward, bodily expression of worship. Part of me wanted to join them, though I was too self-conscious to do so, having been socialized in churches where you stand and sway by your seat and maybe lift up your arms at most to praise God. But I noticed them, and was grateful for their presence.

A few months later at Communion, the side aisles were empty. I found out that the dancers were behind the black curtains on stage, still dancing, but out of sight. My friend Catherine, who led a dance ministry on campus, told me the back story recently. The group had asked to dance at Communion and were given the go-ahead for a while, but then some students didn't like seeing them there in the aisles. It distracted them and made them uncomfortable, they said.

"Distracted," Catherine said, was code for something else. It meant that the bodies of the dancers—all women—by their very existence in the sanctuary, moving in space, were going to cause sin, she explained. Or at the very least, that they were going to keep others from worshiping God. So the dancers were put behind the curtain. They could worship in the ways they felt called, but only out of public view. They were cut off from the rest of the student body, as if what they did was unseemly or even shameful.

The next year, Catherine's group broached the topic again with the chapel worship leaders. She told them, "For those of us who feel we have used our bodies in sinful ways, dancing is an active form of redemption, using our bodies as a form of worship. That's something that isn't supposed to just be for us as individuals behind a curtain, hanging out with God. This is an embodied act of redemption that can be healing for somebody else to see." Catherine's explanation, which seemed so self-evident to her, was a revelation to the worship team. In the end, the group was allowed to dance in the aisles again.

My college, like many Christian communities, had its hang-ups around bodies. We have bodies, but we'd rather not see them. We want to worship God, but we prefer to do so without the "distractions" that our bodies pose. We are the body of Christ, yet we hide those bodies that make us feel uncomfortable, pained, aroused, or threatened, rather than deal with our messy feelings in community. These feelings of shame, confusion, and dissonance between body and spirit also shape our experiences in pain and illness. To understand—and reorient—

our relationship to our bodies in suffering, we need to trace the trail of feelings to their origin.

BEGINNINGS

In ancient Israel, a backwater of the Roman Empire, Jesus' earliest followers proclaimed the news of a man who died by gruesome crucifixion and came back to life three days later, and who then rose into the clouds and promised to come back and make things right. "He was born of a woman, just like us! He said God was his father! He ate fish and broke bread with us after he was raised from the dead! He is coming back to establish his kingdom!"

Listeners found much of it confusing and incredible. That a man who claimed equality with God could bleed and sweat and chew food. That he promised to establish his kingdom, and even said it was at hand, but then died so unvictoriously. Most startling of all was that people saw him walking around and sharing meals after he had so obviously died. As the news spread toward the center of the Empire—the inheritor of classical Greek civilization—the story seemed even more implausible to listeners there, rooted in the thoughts of Plato and his peers. Greek philosophers had little use for the body as anything meaningful or worth noticing. We are living in a cave, Plato said, staring at shadows of the world of perfect forms reflected on the cave wall. The real thing is outside the cave, beyond the body and its shackles.[1] If we can escape the burdens of the flesh and live on a higher plane, then we'll really be free. Sound familiar?

The idea that the body is a secondary, imperfect shadow of our real selves (our souls) wormed its way into Christian thought in a set of heresies we now call Gnosticism. Many of the early church's struggles, and the resulting creeds, such as the Nicene, were a response to Gnostic claims that Jesus wasn't really human or that he only pretended to suffer and die. Even early church fathers, such as Augustine and Gregory of Nyssa, "tried to solve the puzzle created by the full humanity of Jesus set against what is yet unredeemed in our humanity—the painful reality that our bodies don't always act in ways that are healthy, good, or holy," writes spiritual director Tara Owens.[2]

Augustine attempted to root out all sexual desire, since it had been his downfall in his early years, while Gregory of Nyssa figured that our mortality was God's second-best plan, the "garment of skin" conceded to Adam and Eve after the Fall. "Sexual union, conception, childbirth, dirt, nursing, food, excrement, the gradual growth of the body towards maturity, adulthood, old age, sickness, and death" were all part of plan B, according to the saint, and none of it was what God originally intended.[3]

Gregory of Nyssa's ideas might be misguided, but we can learn something by following his instinct back to the beginning, when the first humans were figuring out what it meant to live and breathe in bodies. Much of Christian thinking that deals with the puzzle of our bodies—their sufferings and malfunctions, their sometimes unruly and overwhelming needs and desires—traces the problem back to the Fall. Our bodies were perfect and in harmony with the rest of nature, the thinking goes, but after Adam and Eve ate the fruit, sin entered the world, and with it came suffering, pain, and death. Almost all of our physical suffering—diseases, cancer, and even natural disasters—gets pinned back to that first disobedience that upset the balance of creation. *Why do we hurt? Because we sinned.* That is the takeaway from this common reading of the creation and Fall story. If all our pain can be traced back to sin, it is no wonder that we don't know how to be in our bodies. Everything about them is a reminder of our brokenness and alienation from God, as individuals and as humanity. But is that really the case?

REREADING CREATION AND THE FALL

Are our physical "flaws" like cracks in a windshield, all branching out from that first impact of Adam and Eve's disobedience? Or are there other ways to read the story? I recently talked with Ryan Bebej, a vertebrate paleontologist at Calvin University, about these questions. Bebej told me that in the field of paleopathology—in which ancient diseases are studied through human or animal remains—scientists find evidence of cancer, bacterial infections, and tuberculosis in animals long before humans came on the scene. Which means that disease and death have been around for a while, maybe since the beginning.[4]

Others note that disease and death are built-in mechanisms that serve the balance of the created order. If we didn't have viruses to keep the bacterial population in check, said microbiologist Anjeanette Roberts, "there would be no environmental resources and no ecological space for other types of organisms to live on Earth." Earth would be "one giant ball of single-celled organisms, primarily bacteria," she explained.[5]

The fact that diseases keep populations in check and promote ecological balance is little consolation when you're sick and hurting and can't function. But somehow, stepping away from the idea that diseases are all rooted in the curse of the Fall helps me. If some of what I'm experiencing is part of the natural order of things, I'm more able to accept it, and my body. I don't immediately resist my suffering or wonder if I've done something wrong to deserve it. Even so, I trust this is not the end of the story. Pain, suffering, and death, I believe, won't have the last word when Christ comes again to reign over all creation.

But didn't God issue several curses after Adam and Eve disobeyed the command not to eat from the tree of the knowledge of good and evil? The ground is cursed with thistles and thorns, the serpent is made to crawl on the ground and wage war with the woman's offspring, the woman's childbirth pains will increase, her relationship with her husband becomes strained and complicated, and the man must toil and sweat to bring forth nourishment from the ground (Genesis 3).

Some scholars suggest that these "curses" might be seen more as "pronouncements" of what awaited Adam and Eve upon exile.[6] That is, Adam and Eve's innocent and unharmed existence in the garden might have been a protected state from which they were exiled into the "real world" outside, where the possibility of pain, disease, death, and natural disaster could have already existed. "There was no indication that nature was changed metaphysically after the Fall," writes theologian Richard Middleton.[7] In this reading, Adam and Eve's bodies were mortal, pain was already a normal response for living organisms, and we have always been susceptible to suffering and disease. Perhaps the Fall, rather than *introducing* pain and suffering, made us newly aware of these realities. Irresponsible and destructive human action—sin, as we might call it—likely increased the intensity of these sufferings.

This brings us naturally to questions about God's purposes in making a world that includes the possibility of such great suffering. When there is the chance of genetic mutations that lead to cancer, as well as viral infections and autoimmune reactions that result in a lifetime of illness and pain, how can we trust the goodness of God, or the goodness of our bodies that God created?

Theologian Terence Fretheim points out that God called creation "good"—that is, beautiful, praiseworthy, purposeful—but not "perfect," which would mean without flaw, complete, without a chance for things to go awry.[8] It follows that our bodies, as part of this creation, would also be subject to the same risks, contingencies, and imperfections.

In God's unfathomable sovereignty, he allowed for organisms and natural processes to interact in any number of surprising, unpredictable ways. Weather patterns fuel the agricultural cycles of sowing, tending, and harvest that sustain human society, but unpredictable and extreme weather can lead to drought, famine, and natural disaster. African oxpecker birds eat the ticks off rhinos and water buffalo, but sometimes they also exacerbate the open wounds from the ticks, hurting their hosts.[9] Humans have shorter interbirth intervals than other primates (which can average four to eight years between offspring); this has led to greater social cohesion as families share childcare responsibilities. And yet it also increases the chance of infant mortality, as already limited resources have to be divvied between more children.

It can be difficult to judge whether any natural development is "good" or "bad" in moral terms, and perhaps there is no need to. Our bodies, along with the rest of creation, are good in that God made them, loves them, and has a purpose for us as embodied creatures. Yet they are subject, along with everything else, to what Fretheim calls "wildness": "randomness, risks such as water and the law of gravity, and the potential for ever new developments in the natural order."[10]

This is a different reading of creation and Fall than many of us are used to. There are many loose ends and unanswered questions, unlike the tidier explanation that all suffering resulted from the Fall. But to me, this reading is more honest, making room for the ambiguity we all know when our experiences don't fit into the prevailing narrative, and what appears "bad" at first glance later develops into something "good." This reading leaves room for mystery.

If we accept it, we must reckon with the uncertain "wildness" of our existence, make peace with our limits and vulnerabilities, and learn to live as the bodies we are, with all that we don't know. Certainly, we seek to alleviate suffering. We also recognize that human sin has indeed fractured our relationship with the created order and each other and increased our suffering, in both epic forms like droughts and famines caused by misuse of resources as well as daily forms like alcoholism or domestic violence. It has affected our ability to live well in our bodies and rightly order our desires. Sin has also permeated our human-made institutions, making it harder for groups that have been historically oppressed to be healthy. For example, research around the COVID-19 pandemic, which has disproportionately affected African American communities, shows that it's not just poor personal decisions, but historical patterns of injustice, that make certain bodies more vulnerable to illness than others.[11]

As Christians, we are called to work with God to right our relationships and bring about shalom. But the fact that we have bodies that might cause us pain and suffering has been constant, and we must learn to live—and even thrive—in these fragile vessels.

GENESIS RETOLD

We've briefly considered how the Fall affected our relationship with our bodies, even if it wasn't to introduce pain and suffering. But allow me to creatively retell the first chapters of Genesis to address this more deeply.

In the beginning God created light and dark; water, sky, and earth; plants and stars; sun and moon; birds, fish, and land animals. On the sixth day God sat down at the wheel, took a lump of dusty clay, exhaled moist, oxygen-rich breath onto it, and started to spin. What appeared was a curious little earthen vessel, hard in some places, yet soft and supple; knobby and splayed, yet lithe and nimble; strong and wiry, yet prone to scrapes and cracks; alive and imprinted with God's own image. God called this creature Adam, or "earth," and clapped with delight.

Adam looked about himself, elbows askew, stretching limbs and taking deep, crisp breaths into his newly opened lungs. He spread his toes in the loamy earth from which he came, the molecules in his body recognizing themselves in the ground beneath, a sense of union flowing from toes to fingertips. Crouching, he could feel the juices in his joints compressing and squeezing into new cavities. Then he sprang up, reaching toward the mottled light falling through trees above.

Later, when all the cells in Adam's body yearned to be matched with their own kind, when his arms grasped for the warm body that would exactly fit his, God created Eve, the mother of all the living, and gave Adam and Eve to each other. Together they feasted and explored and nuzzled and exulted in the life and blood that flowed through them. They climbed trees to find the plumpest, sweetest fruit at the top, still warm from the sun. They balanced on mossy rocks in the river, laughing as they lost their footing and splashed into the cool water below. They winced at the scrape, marveling as their bodies reknit the torn skin and flesh.

After the Fall, their eyes were opened. Adam and Eve stared at each other and at their own naked bodies in a strange new light. These tender protrusions—what *were* they? How could they have run and climbed and laughed with each other, with all of *this* so exposed? This could not be right. These soft places, where the blood and energy converged, how could they bear to leave them uncovered, to allow light and gaze to penetrate? In that moment, Adam did not belong to Eve, nor Eve to Adam. They were strangers to each other, and to their own bodies. They were hard, cold observers, noticing the planes and crevices, the rough and the smooth, as liabilities, as points where damage was likely to occur. How could they not have seen this before?

At once, they turned away and looked for covering, for a way to hide these delicate places that spoke to them of their crea-tureliness, their impending death, their susceptibility to forces beyond their knowledge. If they could protect those spots, maybe they could avoid the danger and continue living with abandon. Maybe they could go on not knowing, not thinking, not *feeling* the pain. They reached for the biggest leaves within sight and pulled desperately, piecing together a shield from the knowledge of their own tenuous existence—that it could shatter at any moment, that they could lose everything.

The root of this story, the root of our ambivalence toward our bodies, is fear. Our bodies are uncontrollable, often un-predictable, liable to scrapes and falls, bacteria and viruses, violations and abuse. They always have been. Always will be. They can send mixed signals, and sometimes their needs and impulses conflict with our notions of what is good. Once we realize the extent to which our bodies are not within our control, like Adam and Eve did, we naturally want to minimize the risk. We shy away from that feeling of utter exposure. We cover our physical and metaphorical nakedness. We hide.

TAMING THE MYSTERY

What do our bodies mean? What does our pain mean? What I've tried to show so far is that we often don't know. Being fully human is to inhabit the wild mysteries of our bodies and trust that, because Christ was a body, and still is a body, we don't need to fear this place. We can say, *it is good, because Christ meets us here.*

But this is a complex, uncomfortable space to inhabit. It means we must live in the tension between our susceptibility to pain, disease, and suffering and the truth of Jesus as healer and redeemer. For some, these are mutually exclusive realities. If Jesus heals, we shouldn't have chronic illness, right? Or maybe Jesus still heals, but for people with ongoing conditions that healing is going to be spiritual—that is, we just need to put our bodies aside. Both of these tendencies reflect our innate human desire to make sense out of something deeply confusing, to wrap our minds around something mind-boggling. But in the end, reaching for these tidy answers reduces the complexity in a way that flattens the truth. We end up back at gnosticism or at its opposite pole.

On the gnostic side, the tendency is to make blanket statements that it's all bad. Like St. Augustine or Gregory of Nyssa, we come up against our unruly bodily desires and messy physical functions and simplify by chalking it all up to sin. We lump it all under the category of what Paul called "sinful flesh"

(Romans 8:3) and assume the antidote is to somehow transcend our bodies and to live on a higher (i.e. disembodied) plane. When it comes to illness or pain, this kind of logic suggests that we ignore our pain and bodily discomforts, because they are manifestations of a lower, baser existence, a distraction from our real calling to the life of the Spirit. The tendency toward gnosticism pops up throughout the history of the church.

Ascetic traditions of fasting, for instance, recognized the linkages between body and spirit, that by training our bodies we could influence our spirits. Yet those traditions sometimes verged into gnostic body denial—witness the self-flagellation and refusal to take food by some saints. Catherine of Sienna was one of these, who died at age thirty-three of self-induced starvation, asserting that "true nourishment came only from Christ, and to rely too heavily on earthly food was to commit the terrible sin of gluttony."[12]

In recent decades, many Christians have tried to make sense of the tension between our bodies and spirits by swinging to the opposite pole. Instead of saying, "The body doesn't matter," they have said, "The body matters—in fact—what happens in your body corresponds exactly to what's going on in your spirit." Take evangelical fitness and diet culture, which anthropologist R. Marie Griffith documents in *Born Again Bodies*. Beginning in the 1950s, books like *I Prayed Myself Slim* and *Pray Your Weight Away* inaugurated a wave of Christian self-help literature on weight loss. One author admonished readers, "Stand on the scale. How much more do you weigh than you should weigh? . . . We fatties are the only people on earth who can weigh our sin." He promised weight loss through prayer, devotional Bible readings, and unshakable faith.[13] In the following decades, other authors and Christian diet and fitness programs, like the Weigh Down Workshop, continued to connect spiritual discipline and godliness to thin and conventionally attractive bodies.

In one sense these programs were helpful—they addressed the disconnect between body and spirit and taught Christians to take care of their bodies, which are "a temple of the Holy Spirit" (1 Corinthians 6:19-20). These messages were compelling and motivating—devotional diet books frequently sold hundreds of thousands, if not millions, of copies while faith-based exercise programs spread in churches around the world. Many people did lose pounds and become fitter.

But instead of wrestling with the mystery and wildness of our bodies—the fact that the processes happening within them are often out of our control—Christian diet and fitness programs usually flattened that tension. They conflated bodily health with spiritual health. *If you are healthy and thin, it means God is at work in you, renewing your spirit and your body.* Likewise, *if you are ill or fat, it means you've succumbed to sin. You're not letting God into your life.*[14] As Griffith notes, "the search for external somatic indicators of internal states of being is age-old."[15] That is, we've always had trouble with spiritual uncertainty and tried to ascertain whether we have God's favor or not by looking at our bodies or material circumstances for "proof" that we are blessed, that we are God's elect.[16] The messages from Christian diet and fitness gurus were a subtle manifestation of the prosperity gospel, which, as we'll see later, assumes a neat correspondence between God's blessings and material prosperity. When it comes to illness, prosperity gospel believers respond, *If Jesus is here to heal us, then you'll be physically healed, and if you aren't, then there's some blockage of God's power in your life.*

Both the gnostic tendency of body-denial and the tendency of some contemporary Christians to equate body and spirit are fear responses in the face of the wildness of our bodies. Our bodies are vulnerable, untamable, and often out of our control. But rather than live in the wildness, letting it work on our souls, we try to tame. We dishonor the mystery of our bodies by relegating them to second-class status behind our souls. Or we dishonor them by flattening their truth, trying to make them fit into a middle-class, white Protestant vision of what a holy, "blessed" body looks like.

Our attempts to wrest control show up in other ways. We box in our sexuality with stringent rules around sex and dating, often teaching young people to squelch any sexual desire for fear that it will lead them astray. We buy the latest health elixirs to protect ourselves from the wilds of aging. We bank our children's cord blood as collateral against unknown future illnesses. We build fences around our neighborhoods and walls around our countries to prevent other, darker bodies with their imagined threats of violence and disease from entering. We use so many fig leaves to cover our nakedness.

I don't mean to say that these practices are all wrong, or that we shouldn't try to protect ourselves from harm. But our frantic self-protection keeps us from truly facing our bodies as they are—beautiful, wild, unknown terrain, yet places where God dwells. If we stop being afraid of our bodies, stop trying to simplify the mystery into something we can manipulate and control, we might actually be able to hear what our bodies have to say—whether they are sick or healthy. We might find truer ways to bridge the split between body and spirit. We might heal the fragmentation at the core of our being.

BEING A BODY

I wasn't raised in a Christian family. I only entered the "Christian bubble" of a Southern Baptist youth group in junior high, where I pledged myself to abstinence before marriage at a True Love Waits conference and absorbed other conflicted messages about the life of the body. Growing up in a Chinese immigrant family, though, I wasn't taught to distrust my body or subsume it under other, holier pursuits. If anything, my mother was overly focused on health. "If you don't have your health, you don't have anything," she repeatedly admonished me. Her view reflects the extreme end of the tension we just explored, a tension that theologian Stephanie Paulsell describes as both *being* a body and *having* a body:

> If we believe that we *are* our bodies, we might give greater value to the human body than if we thought it was only the shell that our true self inhabited. But we might also place the fulfillment of our bodily desires above every other consideration, or we might allow ourselves to be defined wholly by our bodies. If we believe that we simply *have* a body, we might resist such constraining self-definition. But we might also come to view the body as somehow distinct from who we are. And we might gradually come to see the body as a hindrance or, at the worst, something to despise.[17]

My mother, who came from a materialist, nonreligious upbringing in Mao-era China, believed that, since we are *just* our bodies, losing health would mean a loss of everything—energy, money-making potential, savings, the future.

This is surely not the best way to live. Yet, because of my mom's body-accepting influence, I was less susceptible to the body-denying messages I later received in many church settings. Growing up, I used the bathroom with the door open, saw my mom dress or undress regularly, and didn't feel large amounts of shame or secrecy surrounding body parts and processes, like having breasts or my period.

I discovered I loved dancing in junior high and high school, which in college and later years became a meaningful way for me to pray and worship. When my church in college went through a dissolution, I led a workshop where we used touch and body movement to process our feelings. One of the participants commented that perhaps if we'd been able to use our bodies to get in touch with some of these underlying tensions earlier, we might have avoided getting to the point of dissolution. I was grateful to be able to lead my fellow church members into a deeper relationship with their bodies and show them how bodies can speak into our spiritual lives.

Fast-forward a few years to when the pain started. Here I was, staring at my tingling and reddish left foot, propped up on a pillow. Here I was again, trying to be cheerful as I crutched around to watch my sister-in-law run the Chicago Marathon, wishing I was not the passive spectator but the active participant. Here I was again, lying in bed with sleep- and tear-blurred vision in my aunt and uncle's house in Changsha, China, while my husband went on a weekend tour of the Zhangjiajie national park. I couldn't go because it involved too much hiking. Being in my body was not fun anymore. I couldn't find meaning and satisfaction the way I used to. *Was* there any meaning to it? It was now hard to affirm that my body was good.

My Christian community supported me, but they didn't offer many resources to live well as the weak, pain-filled body I was now.[18] Mainly, I heard them say, "Just don't think too much about your body. Yes, you are limited in your activities, and yes, you are in pain, but you can still minister and have relationships and grow spiritually. You are okay." This did help, but for reasons I couldn't articulate then, I was still frustrated and wanted something more.

Years later, reflecting on that season, I can finally begin to put into words what that *more* is. I want the church to say, "Your pain is not just something we minister to. Perhaps it is something that can minister to us. We want to learn from your experiences, because the fragility and brokenness of your body can speak to our shared human condition. The suffering you know in your body is something we can all grow from, not something you have to transcend in order to grow." And mostly, I want my sisters and brothers to say, "We see you in your pain. We don't flinch or turn away. It's not unsightly or inconvenient. It's not something we need to solve. Your body is still good. It is still holy. We are with you in your body, just the way it is."

GRASPING AT FIG LEAVES

Unfortunately, Christians don't often receive body-affirming messages from the church in their times of suffering and illness. Because of our gnostic legacy and our tendency to want to squelch mystery, it's easier to fall back on fear, distancing, and blame. In the face of raw, unresolved suffering, we still grasp for fig leaves.

One common fig leaf is trying to find a cause, or a solution. Anglican priest Tish Harrison Warren says this about living with chronic migraines:

> As advanced and broad-minded as we 21st century people
> fancy ourselves to be, there is still something in us—some

silent, gnawing, primordial place in us—that when confronted with unsolvable pain whispers the question Jesus's disciples asked about a blind man: "Rabbi, who sinned, this man or his parents?"

Who, here, is to blame? Of course, this question is now phrased differently. When I talk about migraines, people very naturally want to offer solutions. They suggest therapies that they insist I try (and I often do) or they chastise me for not trusting Western medical treatments enough or for not trying every holistic, alternative treatment. In these dinner-party medical consultations, people are simply trying to be helpful, and I appreciate it. But at 3 am when I'm writhing in pain, the suggestions come to me as accusations: Why can't I fix this? What am I doing wrong? Am I not trying hard enough? Am I just being a wimp?

A friend once asked me if I think too often about migraines and knowingly whispered to me, "I believe that we get sick when we have negative thoughts. If we dwell on something, we make it happen." Am I causing migraines by thinking about migraines?[19]

We want so badly to understand our suffering. If we can pin it down, then we have some control, some way of altering the outcome and covering our nakedness.

If a cause or solution can't be found, another fig leaf we turn to is incessant activity. "If you can't sleep at night, you can pray for others," well-meaning friends might say. Or, "If you can't stand up to volunteer at the soup kitchen, you can at least write letters to prisoners." This isn't bad advice, but underneath it often lies a deep discomfort with inactivity, with the empty, silent spaces where we stare our essential aloneness and helplessness in the face. And when we can't even muster the energy to do these small acts of service due to fatigue and pain, we feel guilty, incompetent, useless. Are we valuable outside of what we do? Can we look with courage at our own weak spots, lingering long enough to get shaken up? We'd often rather not. We'd rather stay busy.

When we see bodies in our midst who don't fit our ideal of spiritual productivity, whose suffering we cannot trace to any particular cause, as a community we grasp at another fig leaf—disbelief and avoidance. Caroline, a woman nearing sixty who has experienced pain and exhaustion since her twenties, speaks poignantly to this. "Fatigue is no joke," she says, "but people think you're making it up. Somebody in the church said to me, 'So-and-so has fibromyalgia—that's a fake illness right? That means they really aren't sick.' Well, I have fibromyalgia. . . . They'd like it better if you said you had heart disease, then nobody would ever begrudge you lying in bed or something."

Overall, Caroline has had an incredibly negative church experience.

I don't even know the point of being a Christian if nobody cares about you when you're sick. Nobody thinks of you. Nobody wants to know you because you might be a little different or you don't feel good enough to be like everyone else or you haven't been as lucky as everyone else. I don't have a husband, children or a house. I'm a non-person. I live in subsidized housing—everybody was grossed out by it. I've had a really shallow church experience. People care more if you break some sort of rule. They'd rather obsess about gay marriage or worry about liberals than loving a sick person in their midst. I feel like a reject.

She wonders if her feelings of dis-belonging might stem from the fact that she's poor and most members of her congregation are relatively wealthy. I think she's onto something. Wealth can be a fig leaf, providing a sense of power over our circumstances. We use it to console ourselves that God approves of us because he has blessed us materially. We fall back on the thought of cushy bank accounts when fear of the future attacks. Caroline's condition—her poverty, her difference, her lack of success and incessant suffering—flies in the face of the stories that many of us like to tell themselves: *God is rewarding me. I've followed the rules, and everything will be all right.* I can "curate my life, minimize my losses, and stand on my successes," as historian Kate Bowler says.[20]

Caroline's very presence in her church is a threat, a needle that would likely burst the bubble of these prosperity gospel fantasies if people paid attention to her suffering. But they haven't. They've avoided her. They don't want to acknowledge their own nakedness, don't want to recognize in her their own human fragility. They distance themselves, they blame her, they fear they might "catch" her suffering. They push her body behind the black curtain, just as my college chapel team did with the dancers. They cover up with fig leaves.

We would all do well, individually and collectively, to examine the postures we hold toward our bodies in suffering, and toward the suffering (or simply different) bodies in our midst. Perhaps we feel shame or guilt because our bodies don't bend to the force of our wills or don't fit into the molds cast by our production-oriented society. Perhaps we feel we should be "overcoming" our pain and compensating for all the time and energy lost to illness. Perhaps we recoil from other people's bleeding, infected, or decaying bodies. Where do those feelings come from? What are we really afraid of?

Our first instinct might be to take action to try to protect ourselves from whatever they have. Or we might distance ourselves and blame them for their pain (with thoughts like, *I'm glad I don't have* that, or *Why didn't they take better care of themselves?*). What stories are we telling ourselves, in these moments? Are they true? Are there other stories or interpretations that might be equally true?

How are we, in our own wily ways, grasping for fig leaves to cover our nakedness? What would happen if we put those fig leaves aside?

3

ELUSIVE HEALING

I sat on a stone bench in a little park near our apartment one September, journaling. It had been about three months since my ankle pain started. Yellow and orange marigolds fanned out in arcs around the paved central plaza, where a tiered fountain invited children to reach in and fish for wishing coins. The sunlight landed playfully on my back and the tree leaves flaunted a green so alive it danced, and you could almost see the chlorophyll being produced. Joggers challenged their muscles, awash in endorphins from exertion; parents pushed babies with fat, wiggly toes in strollers; and creation delighted in its own existence.

I gazed intently, willing some of the beauty to seep into my soul and bathe my body in comfort, but the park seemed a separate world from the one I was living internally. I didn't feel part of the loveliness I saw. Instead, the vitality and movement around me heightened my lack thereof. I was, in the words of Grace, a young woman with chronic migraines, "watching life from the sidelines."

My pain wasn't getting better. I'd seen an orthopedic doctor. I'd tried crutches. I'd tried not walking, then walking. I'd tried

Tiger Balm, heat, ice, kinesiology tape, and elevation. I kept limping back to this park every few days, watching summer melt into autumn as the leaves turned yellow, orange, red, and brown and drifted downward. Here, I spilled my woes into my journal, a jumble of urgent pleas to God, then patience and resignation, then more desperation:

> I'm trusting you, God, for my foot to heal, and accepting a time of rest for my body in the meantime.

> I feel like I'm on the verge of a state of depression. It's hard to get out of bed in the morning and do things because I can't really walk or be on my feet for long. God. Please show me that you're real. Please answer my prayers.

> I am doing all I can to let my foot heal. The rest is up to You.

> I've finally accepted that this injury is going to take a long time to heal, trying to focus on the things I can do and enjoy, rather than the things I can't.

> Here I am again, Lord. What do you want from me? Something feels desolate and parched within me. Restore unto me the joy of your salvation. I long to find a seed of hope in this wasteland of my unmet expectations.

It went on like this for months. I cried out for healing. I bopped around to doctors and tried one treatment after another. I went up for prayer in church, made appointments with prayer ministers, and asked my friends to pray. All I wanted was for things to go back to normal, to the way they were before the pain. Was that too much to ask—to be able to walk?

Slowly, excruciatingly, the months became a year, then two years. I moved through life listlessly, often depressed. I applied and got accepted to graduate school. I attended classes, studied, wrote my thesis, and graduated. I even took a weekend canoe trip with some friends that didn't involve much walking. Sometimes the pain improved, and a little space opened up where I could take interest in the goings-on around me. Sometimes it got worse to where I couldn't sit without discomfort, and the black hole of despair beckoned again. Gradually, though, I got used to having pain all the time and it hummed in the background as I did other things.

By this time, my prayers for healing had changed. For a while, I had just stopped talking to God, much less asking for healing, because it didn't seem to make any difference. When I picked up again, I felt like a different person, and God, too, wasn't the same. I wrote in my journal: "It's odd to say 'You,' God, because it takes effort to acknowledge 'You' as this real person and here-and-now presence who cares and whom I perhaps don't know that well. . . . What is the purpose of praying for my own desires when bad things happen anyway? How can I offer this wound up to You as a weak and vulnerable spot where you can enter?"

My body continued to be a source of perplexity, and not just because of the chronic pain. I started getting acne on my back—a rash of itchy, sore bumps with white tips. Though I was trying not to show it, the stress of graduate school and life with pain took a toll on me, in this case popping up on my skin. I stopped wearing tank tops and made an appointment with a dermatologist, who prescribed me a steroidal ointment that messed with my menstrual cycles, so I stopped using it.

My cycles were another confusing part of my body. My husband and I had been married for three years, and we only used birth control the first year. For two years, we hadn't tried to conceive, but hadn't avoided it either. And nothing happened.

My desire to have a baby grew each month, and I started worrying that maybe this was another part of my body that had gone haywire. I didn't want to approach our possible infertility the same way that I had approached the pain—desperately trying all manner of treatments, despairing when I wasn't "fixed." And yet, I just didn't know—what should I accept, what should I resist and try to treat? To what extent should I try to get my body to cooperate with my intentions? How could I find healing?

MISCONCEPTIONS OF HEALING: GOING BACK TO PERFECTION

It took time, but what I understood as healing changed as the "healing" I prayed for never materialized. My spiritual director recently told me that God answers our prayers in so many ways other than the ones we expect. As I let go of my misconceptions of healing that drove me to desperation, I realized that I was, indeed, already on the healing journey.

My biggest hang-up was this idea that healing was complete physical wellness, like pushing the "reset" button to erase all the bugs and glitches and getting back to brand-new, fresh-from-the-factory condition. The notion came from several sources, both in the church and in popular culture.

In the church, we often think of God's original design for creation as "perfection"—perfect functioning, no illness or pain, everything working just right. However, as we saw in chapter two, there are other ways of interpreting the creation story. Remember Terence Fretheim's note that God did not call his work "perfect," but "good" (Genesis 1)?[1] Within his good intentions for creation, God left room for his creatures to interact independently and for the laws he set in motion to play out in unexpected ways. This is part of creation's freedom, and what enables us as humans made in God's image to partner as cocreators with God, working out his intentions for our thriving in new, ever-changing ways.

Creation, from this perspective, is a work in progress, not a botched-up project that's headed for the dustbin (as rapture and tribulation theology popularized by books like the Left Behind series would lead us to believe). The process of creation, to development, to final destination in the natural world parallels God's work of redemption, church planter Mario A. Russo explains: "A Christian experiences a sudden rebirth called regeneration (origin), followed by a progressively changing life (development), and a final destination of glorification." In other words, he says, creation, like our characters, is being progressively transformed.[2]

We can also take a cue from how God reveals himself in the Bible. God called Abraham out of Ur of the Chaldeans into Canaan, showed up to Moses in the burning bush, and gave the Law to the Israelites. But this was not the full picture. These were layers of a painting of who God is that would not get filled in three-dimensionally until the incarnation of his son, Jesus. Theologians call this idea "progressive revelation"—later books in the Bible give a more complete picture of God than earlier ones. Some, such as William J. Webb in his redemptive-movement hermeneutic,[3] take it a step farther and argue that we need to take the *spirit* of biblical revelation, not just the direct words and cultural equivalents, into account when we apply Scripture in our times. Both in creation and in God's revelation to us, there is a sense of ongoing development.

This means that God isn't always trying to bring the things that go "awry" in his creation back to his "perfect" plan or heal us back to an elusive, nonexistent Edenic state. That kind of God, pastor Bromleigh McCleneghan writes, bears more resemblance to Lord Business in the *The LEGO Movie* than the God she knows. In the movie, the protagonist, Emmet, and a crew of "master builders" try to foil the plans of the evil Lord Business, who wants to "Kragle" (super-glue) everything in place, rather than allow things to be built outside of the directions. Lord Business believes that everything belongs in a particular place. Thus, everything must be built in a particular way, properly ordered and assembled, and if it's not, he'll resort to sinister ends to maintain that order.

McCleneghan observes that, in *The LEGO Movie,* the heroes are "master builders," "individuals who can pull together pieces from a host of different projects or even realms and create something wholly new and wholly useful. Theirs is an ability to envision something no one else would have imagined, and then to bring that vision to birth."[4] She sees God less as "the Man with the Plan" and more like the inspiration that moves these master builders. As she points out, he is the God who invites Abraham to go to a new place, and Jesus asks his disciples to join him in serving. He calls us friends, and no longer slaves. In doing so, God elevates us to the level of cocreators, not just laborers mindlessly carrying out his blueprint.

This understanding of God's world and our role in it has helped me to let go of the desire to "go back" to some idyllic past where I had no pain and things were "as they should be." I certainly grieve my losses. Yet I don't believe that God will push the reset button. And while I also long for something better than this world, a world without pain and suffering, I don't think that it means going back to Eden. Rather, this "better world" will involve transformation, not a rewind, of our pain. The way out is not back, but through.

Just as Jesus took up the cross and turned it from a symbol of shame and punishment to a monument to God's nearness, his oneness with us, so we are called to partner with God and make something new out of our pain. "In the same wound where the pangs of anxiety are seething, creative forces are also being born," writes Brother Roger of Taizé. "And a way opens up that leads from doubt to trusting, from dryness to a creation."[5] Can we sit with our pain long enough to let these forces awaken, rather than wishing the pain away?

Our views of creation inform our vision of resurrection. If we think our created state was perfect, then we expect that our resurrected state will likewise be perfect. And so we view our lives to come through a sugarcoated lens. Will our ultimate healing in heaven result in "the best of the best; glorious, perfectly functioning bodies"?[6] Will we become like newborns with adult bodies, unblemished by the vagaries of life on earth? That doesn't quite fit my experience of God's healing, or the Gospel accounts of the resurrected Jesus.

Luke recounts that, after his resurrection, Jesus appears to his disciples, startling them. They think they're seeing a ghost. "Why are you frightened, and why do doubts arise in your hearts? Look at my hands and my feet; see that it is I myself. Touch me and see," Jesus says to them (24:36-39). He shows them his skin and bones, and his side, pierced by the spear. He is a real, flesh-and-blood person, and his body still bears the marks of his traumatic earthly life. Disability theologian Nancy Eiesland reads in this story part of her hidden history as a Christian: "Here was the resurrected Christ making good on the promise that God would be with us, embodied, as we are—

disabled and divine. . . . Seldom is the resurrected Christ recognized as a deity whose hands, feet, and side bear the marks
of profound physical impairment."[7]

Eiesland's reading might be startling for those of us who
come from an able-bodied mentality, who think of God as su-
premely omnipotent, completely unimpaired. Disabled . . . God?
These words should not go together. Yet her observation is
true: the resurrected Christ was blemished. His body was—
and is—imperfect. His wrists have gaping holes, and the
muscles and tendons in his side are torn and scarred over by
fibrous, white tissue. At the very least, we might conclude that
we will all be, in the resurrection, still profoundly marked in
our bodies by what we have experienced in our current lives,
whether that is cancer or paraplegia or chronic pain.

Many of us yearn for the day when the lame will walk and
the blind will see. But among those who experience profound
impairments, the idea of a "cure" in the life to come isn't agreed
upon. Disability and limitation don't necessarily imply suffering.
Perhaps, as theologian Beth Felker Jones suggests, "all that we
'have survived over the years . . . and been given' is written on
our bodies and is taken up into our salvation,"[8] transformed
into something that we will still recognize as a reminder of
God's presence with us now. Our limitations have shaped our
identity and influenced how we engage with the world and
with God. Would we be the same people without them?

There is no rewinding, no praying ourselves back to a time
when body and spirit were untouched by pain. Rather, there is
wound healing, which involves scarring over, and then therapy
to transform that scar.

At one point in my healing journey, I came across a type of
physical therapy called ASTYM. Therapists work on disorganized,

stuck-together scar tissue by applying a heavy cream and a tool to the area, scraping the scar and dislodging adhesions. On a cellular level, the tool causes microtrauma and encourages the body to lay down new, smoother fibers in a more organized fashion, promoting blood flow and fresh growth. I was squeamish to try it, because up until then my approach had been to leave the pain alone and move my ankle as little as possible. Anyone who has had surgery or been injured knows, though, that while this may be the best approach at first, in time you need to start moving those hurt areas so that they become usable again. Going through physical therapy is painful, but necessary.

I wonder if ASTYM might be a metaphor for how we heal. We tend to the scars. We poke at them gently, maybe even vigorously, when we're ready. Instead of yearning for what our bodies and hearts are no longer (and maybe never were to begin with), we linger in those places of disfigurement and imperfection, waiting for the new growth to appear.

CULTURAL VISIONS OF PERFECT BODIES

There is another problem with our ideas of bodily perfection. They have never been the same throughout history.

I've had the notion for some years now—fueled by trends like the Paleo Diet (large amounts of nuts, seeds, lean meats, fruits, and vegetables, and few grains or processed foods, in imitation of how hunter-gatherers ate)—that our early human ancestors had the ideal conditions for health. They tracked deer and woolly mammoths and gathered wild plants instead of sitting and staring at screens all day and eating McDonald's. They had plenty of leisure time since they weren't tied to the intensive demands of farming. And they lived in a pristine, pollution-free environment. Sounds great, right? Scholars call this yearning for a different time period *historical nostalgia*, "a desire to escape into an imagined, idealized world of a previous era."[9]

As I was doing research recently for an article on the science of aging,[10] though, it struck me that there is nothing nostalgic about primitive human life. Before the agricultural revolution, before microscopes and Louis Pasteur and vaccines, before sterile gauze pads and Neosporin, humans averaged a life span of twenty-five years.[11] An infected cut on the finger that spread to the rest of the body, or the common cold, if it got into the lungs, could spell death. Infants and children frequently died, and if a man or woman made it past childbearing age, they were considered lucky and honored. So even though I think of ancient humans as healthier and more physically fit than people today, the fact is that they were stalked on all sides by potential accidents, illnesses, and death. There was no ER around the corner. Perhaps they were more wiry and nimble, able to climb a tree or summit a mountain much faster than us sofa spuds today. Yet were they living in Eden? Did they have perfectly functioning bodies? I'm not so sure anymore.

Early humans spared little mental energy on getting their bodies into perfect condition through diets, exercise, or supplements. They focused on survival. Today, though, with our medicines and surgeries and health gurus, with slick images of sexy and satisfied women and men everywhere we look, we have lots of ideas about perfection. In today's North American society specifically, the perfect body is slim, young, able, and white.[12] Take almost any major motion picture and identify the protagonists, and you'll find this to be the case.

Things are changing slowly now, as demographics shift and more and more people discover counternarratives to the story perpetuated by white, middle-class folks. Memoirs from people like Ta-Nehisi Coates (*Between the World and Me*) and Roxane Gay (*Hunger*) have become bestsellers, poking holes in the myth that whiteness equals blessedness and purity, and that thinness equals virtue and self-control. These counternarratives help us see that what is considered "normal" now wasn't always considered such. The images we have of bodily perfection have been built up, piece by piece, decade by decade, on the backs of beaten slaves, anorexic models, and anxious everyday people who have leafed the magazines and emptied their wallets, believing the myths. They are lodged not just into pop culture, but also into the medical world[13] and the church.

Other societies and eras have had different images of perfection. In Renaissance Europe, artists like Peter Paul Rubens elevated corpulent women with pale, fleshy folds as ideal. In his painting *The Fall of Man,* Eve has veritable love handles, while in other paintings his Venus has thighs and buttocks that wouldn't fit skinny jeans. Indian women, too, have historically striven toward belly rolls as a sign of wealth and leisure; a bit of jiggle hanging over the sari was a good thing.[14] Even the popular history of the United States in the past century, from the angular flapper women of the 1920s to the busty Victoria's Secret models of recent years, shows that what is "perfect" and "beautiful" changes.

Theologian Joyce Ann Mercer notes that cultural perspectives and norms literally *shape* our bodies.[15] It's not just what we eat and how we move or don't move, but what we desire and value that makes our bodies what they are. "It might seem that something like body shape is a given (we are born with a certain bone structure, etc.), but that would suggest a certain one-way drive between body and culture," she said. "We don't have the body as a given. It is not as if we add culture and stir and get something else. But bodies are shaped by culture because culture is always a part of our bodily reality."

Recent cultural developments in the form of medical advances and biotechnology have further altered what we think of as our normal, given bodily reality. Today, we expect to live to about seventy or eighty in healthy condition. Dying around one's thirtieth birthday—a pretty decent life, to a primitive human—is now a tragedy. We ask what the person could have done (used a seatbelt, eaten all organic, sought professional help . . .) to prevent this disaster. Our newfound abilities to keep people healthy and safe are exhilarating and horizon-expanding, so much so that serious scientists today compete to find the cure for Alzheimer's and cancer and work toward the ability to "have the body and mind of a 22-year-old but the experience of a 130-year-old."[16]

Historian Yuval Noah Harari observes that medicine is no longer just about healing the sick, but upgrading the healthy.[17] He identifies the fine—and fuzzy—line between healing and upgrading. If healing is bringing people up to a "normal," "healthy" condition, but what we consider normal and healthy has changed throughout history, then what is healing? When does it cross into "upgrading"? When are our efforts (and expenses) to manipulate our bodies and their functions justified, and when do they go overboard, reaching for a level of control and transcendence that we were never meant to have?[18]

Fresh out of college, when the pain first started, I derived my idea of "normal" from my peers. The students at my liberal arts Christian college were (and are) some of the most attractive (by mainstream standards) and well-kept human specimens on the planet. Many come from white, middle-class families, work out regularly, wear trendy clothes, and exude an aura of confidence and success. (If you dig more deeply, you'll find we are also some of the most angsty and overburdened college students in the country.)

Upon graduation, my friends were doing graduate work in reconciliation in Ireland, salsa dancing, and taking mission trips to Chad. These, to me, were normal things that twenty-two-year-olds do. When I asked God for healing, what I meant was this: I wanted the ability to once again be master of my fate (or at least have that illusion), to dream something up and have the physical stamina to do it, to return to what my social circle considered "normal," "perfect," and "blessed."

BLESSED ARE THOSE WITH THE RIGHT FORMULA?

Historian Kate Bowler tells of a time when she regularly attended a storefront church that espoused a type of prosperity gospel as research for her dissertation. In the middle of her project, she started getting a mystery pain and weakness in her arms that doctors diagnosed in various ways but treatments didn't improve (I can relate). She would arrive at the church with her arms in splints, acutely aware of being Exhibit A for the congregants regarding what prevents healing: not having enough faith, being subject to a satanic attack, being embroiled in sin, and so on. She writes:

> Sometimes I received an invitation to a quiet room to go over a checklist of sins that I might have committed that would have opened the door to the ministrations of demons with names like Python, Sitri, and Vassago. What or who, my helpers wanted to know, was squeezing the life out of me? They took spiritual inventories, paging through

my life and taking out events one by one for examination. Was this it? What darkness could God's light expose?[19]

For prosperity gospel adherents, life is understood through a set of neat spiritual laws. These laws, Bowler explains, "create a Newtonian universe in which the chaos of the world seems reducible to simple cause and effect. The stories of people's lives can be plotted by whether or not they follow the rules."[20] If you do things "God's way," you will evade suffering, get your healing, and have good health and probably a cushy bank account. These blessings are yours by divine right, if you can only figure out which of God's buttons to push.

This is a laughable caricature, I know, but as Bowler and others point out, we all yearn for this kind of elegantly simple universe in our own subtle ways. When accosted by suffering from out of nowhere—whether the death of a loved one or chronic illness or job loss—we all react with the same indignant, "Why?! What did I do to deserve this? What's your point, God?"

And actually, though we might deride prosperity gospel adherents for their naive understanding of how God works, the idea that "actions have consequences" is quite biblical, theologian Peter Enns writes. He points out that much of the wisdom in the book of Proverbs contains the principle that God blesses the upright—for example, "The LORD's curse is on the house of the wicked, but he blesses the abode of the righteous" (Proverbs 3:33). The history of the Israelites also supports this idea. Before they entered the Promised Land, Moses gave a big speech on how it would work: follow God's laws and enjoy on-time rain, good harvests, and peace in the land, or go your own way and reap disease, drought, starvation, enemy attacks, and misery (Deuteronomy 28).[21]

These biblical teachings prime us to expect certain things from God when we follow his paths. The Bible even seems to make room for questioning and blaming God when our experiences don't match these principles. The speaker in Psalm 73, for instance, says that, though he wants to believe that "God is good to the upright, to those who are pure in heart" (v. 1), he sees instead the prosperity of the wicked, who "have no pain; their bodies are sound and sleek. They are not in trouble as others are; they are not plagued like other people" (vv. 4-5). Other psalms frame God as the main instigator of suffering: "You have put me in the depths of the Pit, in the regions dark and deep. Your wrath lies heavy upon me, and you overwhelm me with all your waves" (Psalm 88:6-7).

The psalmists—and all of us—discover that the world is not so simple as the precept that good people prosper and bad people don't. Yet many of us operate on this assumption and teach our children likewise. We want to believe that our hard work and right choices matter. And they do. What we learn in the course of life, though, is that we've misunderstood "good actions" and "good consequences." "Prosperity," in the fullest sense, might not be what we thought. It's not so cut-and-dried as Bowler's prayer ministers believed, that if you go over this checklist of sins and cross them all off, then your way to healing will be cleared and God's material blessings will flow.

Good actions might not consist in simply following specific formulas or rules but might be, rather, a simple, blind trust in a God who we realize is not quite who we thought God was. It might be continuing to seek God and his kingdom when all evidence contradicts his existence and the kingdom's coming. Good consequences might not be perfect health or an answer to a specific prayer. Instead, we might reap a deep, unshakable peace that God is with us, that we will be taken care of, and that, in the end, goodness and love will reign, whether we have our healing or not.

BEYOND "SHOCK AND AWE" HEALING

In the years since I've had chronic pain and not been healed (at least not in the way I assumed), I've abandoned much of what I previously understood about healing—that it is wiping the slate clean and going back to perfect health or an ideal body, or that it's mine for the asking because I'm one of God's chosen and have privileged access to his power. I've also realized, looking back, that I *was* being healed—*am still* being healed, day by day, week by week, piece by piece, in a slow, painstaking process of taking apart and putting back together. It is a kind of healing that can't happen overnight.

We assume, though, that healing involves an immediate rush of warmth and power, a clear before and after. In a video on the CBN website, Rick Aguilar says, "In that instant, in that moment, I felt warmth in my throat, I felt tingling. But the most fabulous thing was that I felt his presence. I felt his glory. I felt his love. I felt his magnificence."[22] He'd had a growing constriction in his throat for several weeks, but one night as he and his wife watched CBN, he heard Pat Robertson proclaim healing for some viewer with swelling in their throat that made it hard to swallow. "Touch your neck," Robertson said. "In the name of Jesus, be made whole." Then and there, Rick's throat constriction was gone.

Stories like these feed our belief that God reaches down from on high, shoves past the physical stuff, and breaks through in a miraculous, obvious sort of way. But this assumption of

God's "shock and awe" healing, writes theologian J. Todd Billings, paints a picture of a God who is above working through bodies and matter.[23] It assumes that God is the sole actor in history, and that he does all things in a direct, unmediated way, without working *through* people or physical processes. When we think of God as doing all things in our lives directly, without instrumental means, we operate with what theologian Michael Horton calls a "hypersupernaturalistic fatalism"[24]—God does everything, and we just sit back and wait for it.

I see this kind of theology in a friend, who for months believed that God had promised to heal her of cancer and thus refused chemotherapy and radiation because she thought she didn't need it. I also see it in the story of a woman who was healed of her diabetes but went right back to her old, unhealthy eating habits, as if her own actions didn't matter.

I want to hold a space in my vision for God to act in powerful, intervening ways that bypass what we understand of physical laws and human actions. Indeed, the Gospels document Jesus performing physical healings with obvious before-and-afters: a leper is immediately cleansed of his leprosy (Luke 5:12-16), a paralytic starts walking (Luke 5:17-26), a woman stops bleeding (Luke 8:40-56).

I've also heard stories of physical healing from people I know and trust—a friend healed of lactose intolerance, another friend's back pain disappearing, and more. These stories challenge my staid middle-class American Christian assumptions that God doesn't work in those ways anymore. Maybe he doesn't because I don't look for him to. Maybe, because I have so many other resources—access to health care, money, and knowledge of how the body works—I don't *need* to rely on God to work in those intervening, "nothing else to do but wait on

God" ways. I want to learn from those who exercise great faith in God when all else fails. I don't have nearly as many chances to do so in my predictable, protected, suburban life.

Yet it is important to hold those healing stories in context. Physical healing, in and of itself, is not the ultimate goal. When Jesus encountered the paralyzed man who was lowered in a mat through the roof by his friends, his first response was, "Your sins are forgiven." Then, when this provoked the Pharisees and scribes ("Who is this who is speaking blasphemies? Who can forgive sins but God alone?"), Jesus healed the man and told him to pick up his mat and walk—"so that you may know that the Son of Man has authority on earth to forgive sins" (Luke 5:17-26). The physical healing was a means to God's larger end of showing who Jesus was to the world, reconnecting to his people through his Son.[25]

This also applies to the stories of people I know who have been healed. I believe their healings happened *so that* something else might happen. My friend was healed of lactose intolerance *so that* she could then stand on this instance of God's faithfulness as she waited with others. Her own healing pointed her gaze toward the larger truth that God is faithful to us and meets our needs. She could then offer that truth, embedded within the nugget of her own story, to others.

Physical healing is *part of* a larger work of healing that God is doing. You might say that those healings are incomplete. They are part of a process—a deeper, longer storyline that is bigger than our own lives, beyond our place and time. If we only look for God's healing in "shock and awe" ways, thereby sitting back and waiting for him to intervene, we miss the deeper, more lasting kinds of healing that he is working out with us as partners.

PARTNERING WITH GOD FOR HEALING

My own healing, as I understand it now, has involved accepting my body's imperfections and not expecting God to save me from the unpleasant aspects that I can't control. Yet it has not meant giving up and feeling defeated, projecting my current physical state into the foreseeable future, or assuming it will only go downhill from here. I'm all for seeking treatment, for having less pain, more energy, and more mobility. But that is only part of the picture.

When Pat, a woman in her sixties who has had arthritis and fibromyalgia for several decades, didn't experience physical healing right away, it pushed her to desperation and intense engagement with God. That eventually opened the doors to emotional and spiritual healing she wouldn't have experienced otherwise. She's discovered a kind of prayer called Immanuel Prayer, and been "blown away by the tender, amazing, even humorous ways that Jesus has spoken into places of long-standing pain and confusion." Her physical circumstances might not be changing. But, Pat said, "I still feel like I'm moving forward and becoming a more whole person. I don't feel like I'm stagnating."

Yet Pat hasn't stopped going to doctors and physical therapists in the intervening years. She's been peeling back the layers to her fibromyalgia, which include genetic and environmental factors, like food sensitivities. Recently, she happened upon a different combination of therapies that has finally relieved twenty-eight years of agonizing hip pain. "I'm grateful I've kept working on it," she said.

Pat and I talked recently about the tension between pushing for healing versus accepting our current reality. I don't think these postures are mutually exclusive. There are seasons for more of one or more of the other. In my own story, there were times when I had to take a break—for weeks or months—from the emotional stress of going to yet another doctor's visit. Then, eventually, I gathered the gumption to reenter the medical system and try another doctor, another approach.

Others have told me that their physical pain pushed them to address past trauma,[26] adjust stress levels, or consistently practice bread-and-butter preventative measures—sleeping well, eating well, and exercising. These are all ways we partner with God for our healing. We learn to pay attention to how all the aspects of our lives are connected. When something hurts, we turn to the pain and ask, where is this coming from? How can I invite God into this pain? What aspects of my life, my relationships, my habits, my history, is this pain bringing to the surface? (It's important to ask these questions in community, sometimes with professional help.) I might not be able to change the circumstances or remove the pain. But what *can* I do? What *can* I address?[27] The answers may surprise us.

4

THE MYTH OF
MEDICAL MASTERY

*J*ames Novrosky, an orthopedic surgeon, was the first doctor I visited for the pain in my ankle. After cycling through ibuprofen, a walking boot, and crutches with no improvement, he finally ordered an MRI. Even though I'd only been in pain for a couple months, a blip in what would be the grand scheme of things, I approached this test as if it were the holy grail of medicine. *Here, at last,* I thought, *we'll be able to pull back the curtain and see what is really going on.* If the doctor was making educated guesses before, now he was finally tapping into omniscience.

The doctor was the priest, offering me up at the altar of science. The lab tech, robed in her set-apart garments of blue coat and disposable paper booties over her shoes, led me back to the changing room, where I removed my clothing, jewelry, and other trappings of self, becoming instead "the patient"—a sacrificial lamb to be poked, prodded, and scanned by the all-knowing eye of the high-pitched whizzing machine. Then came the ritual offering—the holding still while the machine clicked and beeped, drawing my left leg, secured in an immovable brace, into its innards to be scanned, and expelling me out afterward.[1]

For two weeks, I waited for the oracle to speak, for the final judgment. I was back at the park by our apartment, sitting by the fountain, when the results came in a voicemail from a nurse. I had, Lily said, a "swollen navicular bone." The treatment? Ibuprofen for two more weeks. I put the phone back in my bag, deflated. That was it? I had expected that, by being able to pinpoint the exact issue using powerful magnets and radio waves, by peeling back the layers of skin, flesh, and pain, we would know exactly what to do next. The diagnosis, I had hoped, would be followed by a secret formula—a prescription for a different medicine, a surgery, or some other tool from the priestly kit. And then, of course, I would be healed. This would all be over.

Instead, I was told to do the same thing I'd already done. After a few weeks, I was back at Dr. Novrosky's office. He seemed annoyed to see me, and after some halting questions and a cursory exam, I left. The realization dawned on me that maybe he didn't really know what was going on, despite the MRI. Maybe there was nothing more he could do.

In the next few years, I visited other doctors—podiatrists, chiropractors, acupuncturists, prolotherapists, physical therapists, and more—getting different diagnoses and treatments. With each new doctor, my confidence in medicine's ability to offer the silver bullet to fix my pain decreased. I was like Dorothy in Oz, peering behind the wizard's curtain—over and over. There was no all-powerful wizard here. There was only another human being, well-intentioned but fallible, projecting his voice through the screen of technical expertise.

I'm not trying to say that medicine is an illusion, or that doctors are frauds. Modern medicine has provided very real gains in the past century. We've eradicated or nearly eradicated certain infectious diseases, like smallpox and polio. We've formulated antibiotics and anesthesia. Childbirth is no longer a dreaded, life-or-death ordeal as it was in past eras. Between 1900 and 2003, medical advances have brought the average life expectancy in the United States from forty-nine up to seventy-eight, a 57.5 percent increase.[2]

These advances have exhilarated medical professionals and laypeople. Some medical interventions—such as penicillin, which turned life-threatening infections into minor, easily treated issues—*are* silver bullets, providing quick fixes to readily identifiable problems. But now, after decades of witnessing miracle after medical miracle, we expect that medicine will continue along this exponential trajectory. Since we've added nearly thirty years to average life expectancy in a century, maybe, in the next century, we will be able to live to a thousand.[3] Since we've figured out organ transplants, maybe we'll be able to grow tissue and organs and integrate them seamlessly into an ill person, replacing whatever part or system that isn't working and making them as good as new. Having conquered some diseases, we've taken it upon ourselves to conquer all disease. Chronically or terminally ill people, whose issues don't respond to treatment, come to represent an affront to our technical abilities, poking holes in our inflated sense of mastery and progress.

I speak for many when I say that going through the American medical system has been a fragmenting, disenchanting, and often disempowering experience. Why is this the case? What about the alternatives? How can we seek medical treatment in ways that preserve our integrity and facilitate deeper healing?

PULLED APART IN THE EXAM ROOM

In the stories I've heard and read from people with chronic illnesses, they are rushed through appointments or told to see a different specialist. Their pain is dismissed as in their head. They see multiple practitioners but none have spoken to the others, so they have to explain over and over the reason for each visit, starting from square one. Doctors have different areas of expertise and view symptoms through one particular lens, resulting in sometimes conflicting diagnoses and treatments.

In some stories, though, there is a moment of respite—a pause in the hectic pace and a quiet sigh of relief. It comes when a doctor sits down, holds a person's gaze, and says, "Okay, tell me your whole story, from the beginning." This always surprises people because it departs from the norm of several quick questions squeezed into a fifteen-minute window. People feel, in this moment, that their doctor truly sees them and is listening. Why is this such an anomaly in modern medicine—to feel that your doctor cares?

Rachel Naomi Remen, a former medical professor and therapist to people with cancer, trained as a doctor in the 1960s. In a field of mostly men, she made up for the gender gap by mastering even better than her male colleagues the skills that were valued—"decisiveness, objectivity, competence, judgment, and analytical thinking."[4] Very early in her career, during an internship in pediatrics, she went with her senior resident to tell some young parents that a car accident from which they had escaped without a scratch had killed their young child. She cried with them. Afterward, the resident took her aside and told her that her behavior was unprofessional. "These people were counting on our strength," he said, and she had let them down. She took his reprimand to heart, she writes, and by the time she was a senior resident herself, she hadn't cried in years.[5]

Much later, reflecting on her experiences, Remen identifies what her medical training had done to her. By isolating the left-brained traits of linear, rational thinking, her training cut her off from the right-brained, intuitive parts of herself. Over time, she lost softness, gentleness, and warmth. She lost the ability to function as a whole person, heart and mind connected.

Reading Remen's story, I can finally put into context the expressionless faces of many medical professionals I've seen over the years. This is not how they started out. This is how they were trained to interact. This, they were told, would help patients entrust themselves into their care. When doctors put on their white coat, many also put on a mask that hides the human, feeling parts of themselves. They enter the exam room as Dr. Carter or Dr. Palshikar, the skilled professional who can survey a chart and note symptoms to make an incisive diagnosis and treatment plan. They don't meet their patients as Steven or Ruheena, the man whose daughter has juvenile arthritis or the woman whose healer grandfather took her on visits to the sick throughout the Indian countryside as a child.

There are good reasons to maintain professional distance. Doctors and patients don't have to share life stories at first meeting. Yet, like Remen, I am convinced that the lopsided focus on facts, measurable details, and body parts has done everyone in the medical system a disservice. Patients come to the exam room as a collection of symptoms to be analyzed, leaving behind their stories—the ways they've lived through their illness, their reasons for getting up in the morning and having purposeful lives despite debilitating pain and limitations. Doctors, too, often leave the meaning-making, grieving, hoping parts of themselves behind, fearing that they will muddle their objective thinking. In the process, we lose one of the key ingredients to healing—a sense that we are not isolated, that others are with us, *for us*, in our journey. "Side by side, patient and physician focus on the disease, the symptoms, the treatments, never seeing or knowing each other," Remen writes. "The problem gets in the way and we are each alone."[6]

Separated by a gulf of professionalism, doctors and patients further distance themselves by standing on perceived opposite ends of the knowledge spectrum. Doctors are the ones who have trained for years—they've read the books, seen countless manifestations of the same illness, taken the board exams, and earned the right, we believe, to name the problem and call the shots. In this technocratic vision, patients come to be seen as untrained carriers of this or that ailment. Their experience is partial, imprecise, and unreliable. They are often expected to defer to the doctor's expertise and go along with the program.

There are certainly times to defer to expert advice. During the COVID-19 pandemic, for example, we are relying on researchers, physicians, and epidemiologists to gather the very limited data on how the virus works and tell us what to do to keep it from spreading. We also vaccinate our children because doctors tell us doing so will protect not only our children, but other, more vulnerable people who have immune deficiencies or who may not be able to get vaccinated. In response to critiques that medicine has overstepped its limits, impinging on individual liberties, educator Barbara Peterson suggests that instead of labeling doctors as paternalistic, a

Think, for instance, of the term "quality of life." American psychologist John Flanagan originally formulated the measures for a quality of life scale, separated into categories of material and physical well-being, relationships with others, social/community/civic activities, personal development and fulfillment, and recreation.[9] These categories encompassed many meaningful and important aspects of life, from having a job to having and raising children to helping others. The term has become a common way to measure health outcomes, and is seen as so useful that it has migrated from health care to other industries such as economics and advertising.

The concept comes up regularly in conversations on end-of-life care. As the population ages, health providers are shifting the focus from *quantity* of life to *quality* of life. Kelsey Fitzgerald, a psychology doctoral student, interviewed nearly three hundred older adults on their attitudes toward life extension and found that their view of their current quality of life greatly influenced whether they desired to live longer, given the option of treatments that could extend their life. Those who felt they had lower quality of life had less desire to extend their life. For Kelsey, these conversations were eye-opening, helping her realize, in her late twenties, that it's not how long you live but what fills your life that matters.[10] The concept of quality of life has raised important questions about what makes life worth living, so in that sense, it is a positive contribution from the medical field.

Yet I wonder about the effects of trying to quantify the quality of life. A devastating loss, such as the onset of cancer or the death of a spouse, might drastically reduce one's "quality of life," numerically speaking. Does that mean life is less worth living? Should projections of quality of life be used to determine whether to undertake certain medical interventions?

Perhaps trying to quantify our satisfaction with life and measure "the good life" blinds us to the deeper, built-in urge to live despite all of life's setbacks and sufferings. Perhaps it overlooks the way that difficult experiences can be transformative. Perhaps it makes us forgetful of the primal value of life as sheer gift, not something we add to through our biotechnical skills. In our reliance on medicine and technology, we've often misplaced our hopes in their promises, allowing science to define the good life.

The hoped-for world of transhumanists, who believe that humans can evolve beyond our current physical and mental limitations with the help of technology, is where we're headed if we continue along such a trajectory. English professor Christina Bieber Lake lays out this landscape in *Prophets of the Posthuman*. Previous generations have thought long and hard about what constitutes the good life, Lake writes, and have defined it largely in terms of ethical behavior—treating others well, taking responsibility, and acting justly. Transhumanists, however, have rejected "thousands of years of philosophical and theological thinking about what constitutes the highest and best life available to human beings," instead elevating transcendence and progress through technology above all else.[11] They assume "we inherently know what the good life is (to be free from suffering, disease, death, and other difficulties) and that it is something that we can and must make, not learn."[12]

Lake argues that these prophets of change lead us along a false path, "as if to be healthier, have a longer life, or experience less suffering will necessarily amount to a better life."[13] They keep us striving toward some utopic future instead of loving our neighbors in the present. The same thing happens when we place our hopes singularly in medicine to make us whole, when we grant medicine the sole authority to interpret our bodies and lives.[14] We miss that our healing—and our joy—comes more from how we love and live now than the health we're striving to obtain.

TAKING MEDICINE OFF THE PEDESTAL

I am thankful for medicine—conventional and alternative. After a decade with chronic pain, however, I know that it will not save me. I've recalibrated my expectations and found ways to stay intact and sane in a system not designed with the whole person in mind.

Essentially, I've taken medicine off the pedestal. Doctors, I've realized, are not all-powerful wizards, but finite people operating in a glitchy system. Though medicine aims to heal, that does not mean it will always reach its target. It is, theologian Marva Dawn writes, a "stochastic art." That is, medicine is "not as precise as a science, but instead involves probability and random occurrences."[15] Certain outcomes are not guaranteed. Doctors and other medical professionals also operate with limited time, knowledge, and resources. We have seen this, more than ever, in the time of COVID-19 and medical supply shortages. Medicine has its limits. Knowing this, I can let go of some of my disappointment and angst toward doctors and the medical system.

Since I can't rely on doctors to know everything, I've learned to be my own health advocate and manager, like others I've spoken with. Debi has lived with years of severe pain from interstitial cystitis (or IC, which is also called painful bladder syndrome). She's suffered traumatic experiences at the hands of many doctors. Some told her to stop crying in the office or refused to prescribe pain medication and referred her instead to a psychiatrist. Once, in the vulnerability of being in so much pain, Debi agreed to let a male doctor dilate her urethra before she was convinced of its necessity or adequately informed of potential risks and benefits. It resulted in more pain than she had ever experienced since having IC. She calls it "medical rape." Many feel this powerlessness in the unequal relationship between doctors and patients, particularly male to female.

Debi has had positive experiences with doctors that balance out the traumatic ones. She has also found ways to make her voice heard. For example, she has learned to plan out before appointments what she wants her doctors to hear about her condition, what questions to ask, and what treatment to expect or request. She has figured out what kinds of foods trigger her pain flare-ups and found alternative treatments, such as acupuncture, that make the pain more manageable. In essence, she has moved from being a passive recipient to an active participant in her own care. This could not have happened, she says, without family and friends who validated her pain, helped her find the right doctors, and accompanied her to appointments to help articulate and fill in the blanks of her story.

Debi knows well that healing happens within community, not as an isolated pursuit at the doctor's office. She needs her husband, mother, best friends, and church to be with her in the pain. Sometimes she'll call up a couple of her friends and say, "Alright, my vagina's at it again." Once, she went to Caribou Coffee and started writing about her "weird ass diagnosis": "Honestly, I have a bladder issue that hurts me in my clitoris. Can we just take a moment to laugh about it?" Debi's ability to laugh, along with having people who will listen, has made it possible to continue enjoying life despite crippling pain and depression.

Remen came to recognize this kind of hard work from patients as essential to the process of healing. "Years ago, I took full credit when people became well; their recovery was testimony to my skill and knowledge as a physician," she writes. "I never recognized that without their biological, emotional, and spiritual process which could respond to my interventions, nothing could have changed at all. All the time I thought I was repairing, I was collaborating."[16]

Remen concludes, "We are all providers of each other's health."[17]

WHAT IS ENOUGH?

A few months into the pain, frustrated with conventional medicine, I started seeking alternatives. I went to a chiropractor, who offered to adjust my foot. I sat up abruptly and barked, "No!" The pain had made me that squeamish. So she adjusted my back, which had also started to hurt because of my misaligned walking, and prescribed six weeks of weekly therapeutic massages, which—to my delight—were covered by insurance. She also suggested a food sensitivity test, but since this required a nearly thousand-dollar out-of-pocket payment, I declined.

After the rounds of massage and adjustments, which helped minimally, I tried something more drastic—prolotherapy (also known as nonsurgical ligament and tendon reconstruction). The doctor injected multiple places in my ankle, knee, and back with a dextrose solution that was supposed to inflame the area, triggering a "cascade of healing" and hopefully rebuilding some of the damaged tissue. I did several rounds over the course of weeks, paying three hundred to four hundred dollars each visit. The result: over $1,500 flew out of our bank account and I experienced minimal improvement.

A few months later, I saw a Chinese medicine doctor, who examined the half-moons on my fingernails by the cuticles and intoned, with wide eyes and deep concern, that I have too much fire in my body. He prescribed a pill blend of Chinese herbs—eight capsules three times a day for two weeks—for which I plunked down over two hundred bucks. Predictably, insurance didn't cover this. At home that night, my husband looked up "yin-nourishing foods" and prepared me a meal that included tofu and seaweed to counteract the fire—yang—in my system.

I rotated through more rounds of alternative and conventional treatments as the months went by. The thought grew in my mind—is this expense justified? Should I stop trying to seek a cure and simply live with the pain? I just couldn't imagine only being able to walk a couple city blocks as my new normal.

The fact that I had options—that I even had the choice between pursuing further alternative treatments or not—reflected some of my privilege. My husband's employer provided us with health insurance through a PPO network that allowed me to make appointments with various specialists without needing a referral from a primary care doctor. And while I was exhausting the routes of possible treatment within the network of insurance-covered providers, we had enough money for me to concurrently experiment with alternative treatments not covered by insurance.

Recognizing my privilege came with a sense of guilt, which I know is shared by others with chronic pain or illness who can afford to do something about it. Grace, a college student with chronic migraines, told me she refused to take pain medicine for a period. "I felt like if everybody in the world doesn't have access, why should I?" she said. Pat said her family could have lived in a completely different house than their current

750-square-foot one, if it weren't for her health care expenses for her chronic pain over the decades. "I don't know how to get around the guilt over how much money we've spent," she said.

I have circled through the guilt with a mixture of gratitude for the resources I have and anger and lament over the injustices built into our society. I don't have hard and fast answers. Each health care decision requires a separate act of discernment. I have noticed, though, looking back at my own patterns of decision-making in the early years, that I often approached treatments with a sense of desperation. "I'll try anything; I just want to get better!" When it comes to my children's health, too, fear of very rare risks or worst-case scenarios sometimes gets the better of me. My husband, with his engineer's mindset, walks me back from the fear and asks questions that have helped us consider individual health care decisions within a larger context. These questions include:

- What is the cost (in terms of money as well as time and energy)?
- What are the chances that it will work?
- How much will our life improve if it does work?
- Would undergoing this treatment bring more stress than the problem itself?
- Are there other ways we want to use this money, time, or energy, that would give us an equal or greater level of benefit?
- What if we didn't do anything? (Engineers are trained to also weigh the costs and benefits of the "do nothing" option.)

Matt has had his own health issues, suffering from insomnia for extended periods. At one point he sought help from a natural medicine doctor, who recommended removing certain foods from his diet. He did this for several months and didn't see any changes to his sleep patterns. Though he could have continued with this treatment, he decided to change course. The stress of avoiding those foods and figuring out what he could or couldn't eat, along with being hungry and fatigued all the time, outweighed, to him, the potential benefits (the chances of which he questioned at this point).

By contrast, my friend Kimberly has experienced significant relief from her fibromyalgia symptoms by changing her diet. It means she has to bring separate food with her everywhere and that her family's food bill has grown. At points, she thought, *This is too much management. Let me just eat whatever I want.* But her body was "hanging on by a thread," and eating those restricted foods made her "feel like hell all the time." She has been coming to the conviction, with her husband's full support, that she needs to buy the foods that keep her body feeling well, even if they make up a disproportionate amount of their food bill. It doesn't do her—or her family and neighbors—any good, she said, if she's starving because she's unwilling to spend money on the pricier food she needs, or if she's in pain from eating foods that trigger flare-ups.

Early in the chronic illness journey, when we don't have a diagnosis and are visiting different doctors with different approaches, the questions my husband poses are much harder to answer. We're desperate to get relief. We don't know how much improvement a treatment will bring. The chances of success may be unclear. We don't know if a treatment will be more painful than it's worth. But we should ask doctors pointedly for their best guesses at answers to these questions, so we know exactly what we're consenting to.

For me, it was crucial to have my husband as a partner, even after I decided to undergo a treatment. He kept asking questions, such as, "Is this actually working, or are you still doing this because you are desperate and scared?" and "What are your other options?" I needed minds besides my own working on the problem—people who weren't so mired in pain and fear who could help me see a bigger picture. Kimberly, too, needed her husband's involvement, in her case to affirm that what she was doing *was* working, and to give her his full blessing to take care of herself. We need community to help us problem-solve, to see our own heart postures and blind spots clearly, and to find a way forward.

MY HEALTH IS YOUR HEALTH
(AND VICE VERSA)

Kimberly came to terms with the money and effort that treating her illness required by realizing that she could only attend to the needs of her family and the world if she also tended to her own needs. Her needs are important. Her husband's and children's needs are important. Her neighbor's needs are important. None are more important than the others. They all equally deserve attention. Meeting those needs may require different amounts of expense and different allocations of resources. We don't need numerical *equality* (everyone gets the same share) in order to have *equity* (everyone gets their different needs met so we all have an equal chance at thriving in this world). We also don't need to feel guilty for having things that we believe everyone in the world should have—clean water, decent health care, access to pain-relieving medicines, nourishing food, and so forth. But we should certainly work toward others having those things we think everyone needs.

Those of us who have experienced chronic illness may be in a better position than most to see what equity—justice—really requires. We have been on the frustrating receiving end of inadequate health care—care that focuses on tests, numbers, and body parts rather than the lived experience of a whole person within a community. We've been harmed by the current system. We can name the ways it has failed people who are vulnerable.

In addition, our awareness of the ways we have benefited from safety nets, relationships, education, and knowledge—resources that have helped us compensate for what illness has taken—and even our wrestling with guilt and privilege, can turn us toward others. We know not everyone has these resources. From this angle, we can begin to build bridges with other underserved groups—racial minorities, people with disabilities, women, and immigrants, for instance.

Having struggled with the questions of what we need, what is enough, when to push, and when to stop, we can translate our hard-earned insights to the larger, thornier issues in our health care systems. For instance, we can join theologian Stanley Hauerwas in asking questions like, why does a ninety-year-old receive a heart transplant that costs hundreds of thousands of dollars while children die of treatable pneumonia?[18] What does each person in society need in order to thrive? Are we letting fears of death drive us, rather than concern for life?

We can also offer an important rejoinder in the health care conversation by how we define health itself. Instead of seeing a higher "quality of life" or the absence of disease as the standard, we can reframe health as *shalom*, which, notes disability scholar John Swinton, is the closest word for "health" in the Bible. Its root meaning is *wholeness, completeness,* and *well-being.* "Shalom is not the absence of illness, disease, or disability. It has to do with the *presence* of God," Swinton writes. "*Healing always has first and foremost to do with connecting and reconnecting people to God.*"[19]

We can ask ourselves, as we care for our bodies and engage in broader conversations around health care policies, what will bring us closer to *shalom*. How can we stay connected to God and others? What fears or illusions of control are driving our decisions, and how can we relinquish these to God? How can we be present to our own pain and needs, and how can we then translate that tender care to how we relate to our neighbors, and even to the rest of creation?[20]

These are crucial questions, because our well-being is linked to the well-being of others. We are stewards of each other's health, particularly the most vulnerable in our midst. Health, physician Bob Cutillo says, is not a possession to be hoarded, but a precious endowment to be nurtured and shared.[21] I cannot pursue my illusion of keeping my children uncontaminated by environmental toxins without realizing that the very air they breathe and the water they drink is shared by all children. I can spend all my money on masks and immune boosters to prevent my own family from getting COVID-19, but my life in community will be diminished if I don't also care for my neighbors who have lost jobs, and for older adults who are afraid of going out. We are connected to each other in countless, invisible ways. "We are," Eula Biss writes, "continuous with everything here on earth, including, and especially, each other."[22]

Health care is much bigger than me taking care of my own family or seeking the improvement of my own pain, though it may start there. Neither is it just about doctors mastering the scientific knowledge to fix all our problems. Health care, in the end, is about all of us understanding our connection to our families, our next-door neighbors, and our global neighbors, not to mention to the rainforests in Brazil and the penguins in Antarctica. It is about tending to the ailments right in front of us and seeing their relationship to the ailments of our society and our planet. It is being able to pursue healing on individual, interpersonal, and structural levels, knowing we cannot tend to one without tending to the others.

5

THE BURDEN WOMEN BEAR

"For a woman to admit she's in pain puts her in a more vulnerable position than a man who is in pain," said Joy, a woman with fibromyalgia. Joy knows this from not being taken seriously in medical settings and in everyday life.

When she worked as a nanny during the onset of her illness and had to request sick days, she would get the response, "Do you think you can just come in anyway and work while you're sick?" This came primarily from the father of the family, who worked from home and was the parent she most often interacted with. On her last day working with this family, she told him, "I just tried to lift the baby off the changing table but I got really dizzy. I'm not safe to take care of your child." He said he would call a backup. An hour later, with no backup in sight, the mother of the family returned and saw Joy struggling to carry a load of laundry upstairs. "You look really sick. You need to go home," she said.

"If I were a guy it would've been harder to admit," Joy surmised, "but if I'd said it, I think I would've been taken seriously." This refrain of having one's pain dismissed or minimized was repeated over and over by the women I spoke with who live with chronic illness.

WOMEN'S ILLNESSES:
MISUNDERSTOOD AND MINIMIZED

How a person experiences illness and pain differs based on their gender (as well as their race and other socioeconomic factors). Women experience "invisible illnesses" (chronic illnesses that are often hard to measure, diagnose, and treat due to their multisymptomatic and changing nature) at higher rates than men. Over 75 percent of people suffering from autoimmune disorders are women. These disorders include lupus, Sjogren's syndrome, ulcerative colitis, rheumatoid arthritis, and thyroid disease, among others.[1] Women also report pain and chronic ill health at higher rates than men.[2] While this is partially explained by women's tendency to be more willing to talk about health issues and seek more social support, research has also found clear biological differences in the ways women and men feel pain. These include differences in reproductive hormone levels that mediate pain, different genes for stress-induced pain-relieving responses, and differences in central nervous system regulation.[3]

Even as some researchers conclude that women have "enhanced pain sensitivity" and different, perhaps more complex, health care needs than men, women are routinely undertreated for pain. Studies show a marked health care bias against women: women's complaints are dismissed as "in their heads," and assumptions abound that women "have a natural capacity to endure pain" while men are seen as needing more help getting over their pain because they are the breadwinners. Thus, women are more likely to be given sedatives for pain while men are given pain relievers.[4] In one fascinating study male and female students were asked to guess pain levels for low back pain patients based on facial expressions. The patients (15 male and 13 female) had previously been rated by a separate panel of male and female judges on a scale of attractiveness. The researchers found that perceived attractiveness didn't affect the judgment of pain intensity for male patients, but female patients seen as unattractive were more likely to be perceived as experiencing greater pain, while female patients seen as attractive were more likely to be viewed as able to cope with their pain.[5] Given that our current medical system is still male-dominated, the fact that attractiveness could affect the assessment of pain—and thus the level of treatment—for female patients is worrisome.

Many of the women I spoke with expressed a sense of frustration, voicelessness, and extreme vulnerability when navigating a system insensitive to their needs. "I have learned to be tougher. I do my best to not cry. People are not taken seriously when they're crying," said Debi. "That is misleading. If I come in and I seem like I am fine, are they supposed to believe me?"

Anthropologist Emily Martin has explored women's medical experiences through the lens of pregnancy and labor. Analyzing the ways women talked about their prenatal and childbirth care, she found that women often see themselves as passive recipients, with treatments and interventions being "done to them." Obstetrical and childbirth preparedness texts, Martin writes, see the uterus as an involuntary muscle. This perception goes back to nineteenth-century assumptions that women were controlled by their ovaries and uterus: "The female was pictured as 'driven by the tidal currents of her cyclical reproductive system.'"[6] Hence, we get the word "hysteria," coming from the Greek root *hystera*—uterus. In other words, women can't be trusted—either in our self-reports of pain or in being part of medical decisions. We are, apparently, too overcome by bodily forces to think rationally. Christians, particularly, can promote these beliefs. One writer recently called PMS (premenstrual syndrome) a "monthly fight with the flesh,"[7] as if our hormones were our enemies.

Women, like racial minorities, people with nonconforming sexual identities, and people with disabilities, are a vulnerable group. We have different needs because of our biology—particularly our ability to grow babies in our wombs. And while our bodies' uniquenesses may have been designed by God as a blessing, human societies throughout history have turned bodily difference into a reason to devalue our bodies and render us more socially limited, more "tied down." A hierarchy of rank has developed, with bodies that don't conform to the ideal (which has typically been lighter-skinned, male, able, and heterosexual) seen as inferior, exploitable, and even despicable.

What do we do with our differences, which are so vulnerable to abuse? What do we do with the sad fact that women's bodies have consistently been violated, ignored, misunderstood, and devalued—specifically when it comes to chronic illness?

Partly due to biological facts, and partly due to cultural interpretations, women have no choice but to pay more attention to our bodies. This physicality—this vulnerability—has often been a burden. It may also be our greatest strength. The bodies of women and people in other marginalized groups don't have to be prisons that we seek liberation from in order to arrive at our "true selves." Instead, the ties to our bodies can bring us home, bring out our better selves. When we model healthy embodiment, we can lead others who are most distant from their bodies toward wholeness.

BEYOND BODILY ESSENTIALISM
OR CONSTRUCTIVISM

Why *do* women have "invisible illnesses" at higher rates than men? Why is the medical system so biased against women? Are women really just weaker and more prone to hysteria and overreaction, as many health care providers seem to assume? Have we succumbed to the "tidal currents" of our bodies, instead of transcending them with our rational powers?

The last two are trick questions, of course, because they operate within the binary framework so prevalent in Western thought. This framework assumes a set of dualities:

Male	Female
Soul	Body
Mind	Body
Culture	Nature
Public	Private
Reason	Intuition[8]

These dualities are set in opposition, as if what is bodily cannot also be soulful, or what is feminine is automatically irrational. As many feminist thinkers have noted, these are false dichotomies that don't reflect the complex, multilayered realities of our lives, but they have been wielded to sanction a kind of "natural order" where "attitudes and actions toward all that is bodily are closely coordinated with attitudes and actions toward women," theologian Beth Felker Jones writes.[9] This order ranks feminine, bodily things as inferior.

For many of us, Christian instincts (rightly) point to the truth that we are all—women and men—made in God's image, equal before God in value and purpose. The Christian story also highlights how much God values our bodies through coming in the flesh in Jesus. So how do we address the ongoing problem of women and their bodies being seen as inferior? This is the point on our journey together where the terrain gets thorny. Potential landmines lie everywhere. I hope you'll stick it out with me to the end.

An earlier generation of feminists (liberal feminists, they are called), wanting to elevate women to the same level as men, attempted to do so by dissociating women from their bodies. If women's unique association to the body has been problematic, let's cut the ties, they said. Bodies aren't important. Women are equal with men because they are also rational and can participate in the public sphere. Women are no different than men. This move, however, continues to perpetuate the dualism of mind and soul versus body. It also neglects the real bodily differences and needs (such as maternity leave) that women have.

Post-liberal feminists made some different moves. Many have tried to deconstruct the body entirely. Philosopher Judith Butler, for instance, argues that gender is a repetitive act which "reenacts" and "reexperiences" socially established meanings. In other words, gender is not tied to biological necessities and is "real only to the extent that it is performed," she writes.[10] These kinds of theoretical moves deny that bodily facts have any tie to gender and its cultural meanings. They are constructivist, in that they perceive gender roles as socially constructed, rather than biologically determined.

Some Christian circles I've been part of, in response to feminism, have made opposite moves, seeking to elevate women by revaluing their bodies. Women and men find purpose and worth, they say, precisely because of their biological differences. Women can understand God's purposes for them through taking cues from their biological functions—the capacity to carry and nurture babies translates into the overarching "feminine" gifts of receptiveness, openness to life, hospitality, and caretaking.[11] In contrast to post-liberal constructivists, these Christians place meaning precisely in our physical makeup. They are essentialist in the conviction that we can discern some core, essential qualities about "womanhood" or "manhood" by generalizing upon our physical differences.

I want to map out this tricky landscape in advance,[12] because in addressing the question of why women have higher rates of chronic illness than men (and what to do about it), it can be easy to fall into essentialist or constructivist traps—to say "Oh, women are just more physically susceptible to getting sick" (read: weaker) or "It's a problem of male-dominated social oppression." The reality, I believe, is a complex mix of physical and social factors, of bodily tendencies and cultural meanings. Our biology is not our destiny, but neither are our bodies blank slates on which we can write anything we please.

Complicating matters further, we have to discern which of our physical tendencies are "natural"—or God-intended—and which are subject to our fallen condition (for example, some Christians take traditional gender roles to be God's original design, while others read them as patriarchal results of the Fall). "Not only has our access to nature been questioned, but we have also come to realize that those things we have called natural have been marshaled to sanction our own sinful desires," Jones writes.[13] Keeping this fraught terrain in mind—and acknowledging an overlapping spectrum of possibilities rather than polar opposites—we can explore the factors affecting women's health without falling into false dichotomies.

STRUCTURAL INEQUALITY'S
IMPACT ON WOMEN

Shalon Irving was a single black mother who knew all about gender and racial disparities when it came to health. With two master's degrees and a double PhD in sociology and gerontology, she worked as an epidemiologist at the Centers for Disease Control and Prevention, studying how structural inequality, trauma, and violence make people sick. She entered her first pregnancy at age thirty-six with her eyes wide open, aware that her status as a black female made her doubly vulnerable to poor health outcomes. So she assembled a network of "sister friends" around her, steeped in research about how social support could buffer against stress and adversity. Yet in January 2017, three weeks after giving birth to her baby girl, she collapsed and died from complications of high blood pressure. All her education and social support did not protect her against becoming part of a troubling trend—black women in the United States die at three to four times the rate of white women from childbirth-related causes.[14]

One of the biggest causes for this gap, as the NPR coverage on Irving's story explores,[15] is stress. Black women—no matter their level of education or income—live their lives constantly fighting a system that works against them. From the beginning, they struggle uphill in communities with fewer resources than white counterparts in terms of good jobs, reliable transportation, healthy food and safe drinking water, safe streets, and good schools. When it comes to medical care, black women experience even greater disrespect and discrimination than women in general. "It's chronic stress that just happens all the time—there is never a period where there's rest from it. It's everywhere; it's in the air; it's just affecting everything," Fleda Mask Jackson, an Atlanta researcher studying birth outcomes for middle-class black women, told NPR.[16]

Ongoing, unrelieved stress can have a terrible effect on our health. Arline Geronimus, a public health professor, coined the term "weathering" to describe stress-induced wear and tear on the body. She found that, at a cellular level, black women age more quickly than white women. At ages forty-nine to fifty-five, for example, their telomeres (chromosomal markers of aging) were 7.5 years "older" biologically.[17] The result for black maternal health? Black mothers are 49 percent more likely than white mothers to deliver prematurely and more likely to experience pregnancy-induced complications like preeclampsia and high blood pressure.

I mourn for Shalon Irving and her mother, Wanda, left to care for Shalon's baby girl, Soleil. Living in a society not structured with our interests in mind wears at our bodies, making us even more vulnerable to health risks. Because Shalon was a black woman, she experienced this beating even more than nonblack women. And since we all live in this same society that gives preference to men and often exploits women, it makes sense that women experience more invisible illnesses, more pain. All of us are stressed from our uphill battle.

In fact, women are twice as likely to suffer severe stress and anxiety as men, one study finds.[18] And research has now established tentative links between the onset of some autoimmune disorders and stress.[19] Another part of the structural inequality that contributes to stress, one reporter suggests, is women's shouldering of more unpaid domestic work and emotional labor than men.[20] Sociologist Arlie Hochschild calls this double burden of childcare and housework, in addition to work outside the home, the "second shift."[21] These burdens, and the sense of always having to prove the value of our work, our bodies, our very existence, take their toll on our bodies in myriad seen and unseen ways. Sometimes, as we discover years later, they show up as chronic illness.

BODY BURDENS: TWISTED AND REDEEMED

I don't believe the relationship between women's health and chronic illness is solely defined by culture or nature. It's some of both. The way our society operates shapes how women experience our bodies and our potential to thrive. Yet, that is not the end of the story. There is also the actual fact of our bodies.

Throughout history, women have often been deemed more physical, fleshly, and bound to our bodies than men. We have monthly menstrual bleeding, leak milk, and have this tendency to house other bodies within our own. Our bodies are not tidy or easily contained, and perhaps for this reason women's bodies have been feared, labeled as Other. Feminist scholar Donna Haraway notes the problem of bodily divisibility for women: "That, of course, is why women have had so much trouble counting as individuals in modern Western discourses. Their personal, bounded individuality is compromised by their bodies' troubling talent for making other bodies, whose individuality can take precedence over their own."[22] And yet, while women's reproductive powers have indeed been used to diminish our humanity, these same capacities have simultaneously been elevated to an ethereal and otherworldly level. Consider the deification of Mary, the mother of Jesus, in Catholic circles or the characterization of mothers in the Victorian era as "beneficent, chaste, pure, asexual, nourishing."[23]

Poet Adrienne Rich sees the denigration and deification of women as two sides of the same coin of patriarchal mythology. "In order to maintain two such notions, each in its contradictory purity, the masculine imagination has had to divide women, to see us, and force us to see ourselves, as polarized into good or evil, fertile or barren, pure or impure."[24] Again, we come against the false dichotomies of Western thought. Must we deny our connection to the physical in order to function as full-fledged members of society? Must we flee our bodies themselves in order to escape the negative labels attached to them?

As I write, my waistline is planetarial from seven months of growing a human being within. I didn't plan for this one, as I did the other two. The discovery that I was again pregnant came after my husband and I had decided that we were done having more kids, after I had sold or given away most of the infant clothes and looked upon the newly empty spaces in my closets and schedule with satisfaction. With this third pregnancy came the barrage of familiar angst that kept me company in the infancies of my older sons: *Why me, and not my husband? I didn't choose to have breasts or a womb, yet here again I am bound to the needs of a completely helpless tiny human, who relies solely on me for nourishment. Couldn't God have found a more equitable way to distribute the labor (literal childbirth labor too!)? Maybe if men had breasts at least they could fulfill that end of the deal?*

As a woman, my intense awareness of my body and the needs of my children can often seem burdensome and unwelcome. I sleep lightly through my babies' infancies, waking up to their slightest whimpers (or the ghosts of their voices in the form of sirens and cat howls). My husband may sleep through rounds of louder crying. My breasts leak when I hear their cries, and I cannot go too long without nursing (or at least pumping). This pregnancy, I've developed gestational diabetes, so I've had to track my blood sugar and carbohydrate consumption. These are all undeniable physical ties, things that my husband—bless his dear heart—doesn't deal with.

Am I socialized into some of this bodily awareness, this sense of responsibility? Perhaps so, in the same way that women are twice as likely to be the unpaid caretakers of chronically ill people,[25] and in the same way that women shoulder most of the unpaid domestic work and emotional labor. Yet the biological links persist. A woman's heart rate and brain activity increase at the sound of an infant's cry, priming her to respond rapidly.[26] Breastfeeding produces oxytocin, a neurochemical that promotes bonding between mother and baby.[27]

On some sleep-interrupted nights, I'd like to escape from my body and its ties, to ignore my dripping breasts and my pounding heart, to disconnect from the entire baby-body business. At the deepest level, however, I want to believe that leaning into these ties is what will bring me back to my better self, to connection with others, to wholeness. I don't want to turn away from my children, but toward them. I want to do so in a way, though, that does not negate my own needs for rest, nurture, and creative expression. I want to express and meet my own and my family's whole-person needs in a community of other whole people relying on and caring for each other, attending to our weakest members.

No, an escape from the body isn't what's called for in order to liberate women from an oppressive system that harms our health. What's called for is a return.

TURNING TOWARD OUR BODIES

Women's bodies—our vulnerability, our sensitivity to pain, our heightened awareness of others' needs—have been used to violate, exploit, and diminish us. But the way to redemption and wholeness is not to escape; rather, it's to turn these very vulnerabilities into strengths, to stay present to the pain, to see what new growth the wounds might bring forth.

As a young woman, Dorothy Day lived a bohemian life with other intellectuals and social agitators in New York City in the 1910s and 1920s. During this period she had an abortion, which left her traumatized and heartbroken. At the time, she was caught up in the whirlwind changes of her time, in love with a man who couldn't care less about her pregnancy. "It never occurred to me," she would say in her eighties, "to keep the baby." Perhaps it was unthinkable, in that moment, to be weighed down by her pregnant body and its ties without social support.[28]

A few years later, after she thought she was sterile, Day was elated to find herself pregnant. This time she carried her baby to term and birthed her daughter, Tamar. As she embraced motherhood, she also discovered the Catholic faith. In 1938, she went on to found the Catholic Worker Movement with Peter Maurin, which is focused on service to the poor and which came to include "houses of hospitality," where "'countless thousands have been sheltered,' 'millions of meals have been served,' and guests and workers share life together."[29]

Day didn't say so herself, but reading her story, I wonder if her ability to stay present to her bodily limits by offering hospitality to her second unborn child directly fed into her later work of offering hospitality to countless vulnerable people in the Catholic Worker Movement. The movement has become the spiritual grandparent to many other movements and ministries, including the L'Arche communities, where "people with and without intellectual disabilities live and work together as peers."[30] Perhaps Day's "wound where the pangs of anxiety are seething" was her accepting the vulnerability of motherhood, being a female body that could conceive another human being. By living into that wound—grieving her abortion and welcoming her second child—she might also have tapped into the deepest resources of her spirit, the "creative forces" that would lead to a worldwide movement seeking justice and offering hospitality to the poor.[31]

Beth Jones imagines that the bodily differences that have been used by so many male-dominated societies to oppress women will be redeemed by God in our bodies, not away from them. "The gender bending of sanctification, both now and at the eschaton, can only be *toward* care of the body. Living the gendered body, when ordered toward God, might be especially about care of the bodies of the vulnerable," she writes. "If this looks less like masculinity, as we have often known it, and more like that traditionally despised bodily femininity, we should not be surprised. God uses the weak things of the world to shame the strong (1 Corinthians 1:27)."[32]

PERMEABLE TO GOD

Historian Lauren Winner recalls reading Isaiah for an Old Testament class in seminary and being stopped cold by the image in Isaiah 42 of God as a laboring woman. She immediately pictured a grainy black and white photograph from the feminist 1970s of a woman in a hospital bed, "her long, blond hair tied back from her face, her right hand on her forehead, a nurse's hands on her engorged stomach, her face knotted in agony.

Although it was a photograph, you could practically hear a low, loud groan emerging from her throat."

Winner was profoundly disturbed and uncomfortable imagining God laboring like that woman. Or imagining God in the other female roles of midwife and nurse that Isaiah uses, as she later discovered. Yet, these images compelled her, and she pushed into her reaction of "wild unease" to explore what they said about God and God's work: "I realize that my own discomfort includes not just theoretical worry about a God's vulnerability but fear of my own vulnerability. Isaiah's picture of God suggests that those moments when I stop fighting my own vulnerability are exactly the moments when I most participate in God's very nature, in God's very life."[33]

Yes, and amen. And yet. The vulnerability of childbirth is quite different from the vulnerability of chronic illness. A laboring God is still a God bringing forth life. Can we imagine God joining in our sickness, in our nights of troubled sleep and unrelenting pain? What good—what life—does that bring forth?

We might take a clue from Haraway's expression of our problematic divisibility, our bodies' unwillingness to stay within the lines, our bodies' penchants to let our boundaries be crossed. *Permeability* is a good word for this. The first definition Google gives is "the state or quality of a material or membrane that causes it to allow liquids or gases to pass through it." Women allow blood and milk and babies to pass through us. We allow others' needs to touch us, move us to care. We are permeable. Perhaps, too, our permeability makes us more susceptible to certain illnesses, including autoimmune disorders.

Intriguingly, a recent paper by medical professor Vaishali Moulton supports this idea.[34] In humans and most vertebrates, females take on the task of bearing offspring. Female hormones, like estrogen and progesterone, control the reproductive system, but they also regulate the immune system, stimulating a heightened immune response. This response could be crucial, Moulton writes, to a process called "transgenerational immune priming"—that is, the passing on of immunity from one generation to the next through nongenetic means. In humans, mothers pass on antibodies to viruses and bacteria they have already been exposed to through the placenta and in their breastmilk, "priming" their children to fight infections.

In other words, women may have heightened immune responses because they are the half of the species that bears offspring. In some fish species, where the father carries eggs to gestation, there is evidence that males have heightened immunity during the parental stage, Moulton writes. A heightened immune response means that women may be able to fight off acute infections (like influenza[35]) more easily than men, but sometimes after the infection is over the immune system is still in overdrive, resulting in autoimmune disorders. Women's permeability—in bearing children, in passing along antibodies to those children—increases our susceptibility to chronic illness.

Even here, God joins us, as doctoral divinity candidate Julie Morris explores in her reading of Jesus' encounter with the hemorrhaging woman (Mark 5:25-29).[36] To set the scene, Morris explains that in the first century, the body's vulnerability to disease was a gendered reality: "Females were perceived as porous, lacking boundaries between the body and the exterior world, which left them susceptible to illness. The fact that women menstruated monthly demonstrated their inability to control their body or protect it from external forces. In short, a leaking body was a feminine body, an inferior body."

The woman who approaches Jesus in Mark's story has been bleeding for twelve years. If leaking is a bad thing, this woman is worse than most. She can't even contain her bleeding to a few days of the month. When she touches the fringe of Jesus' cloak, something unexpected happens. Jesus feels the power go out of him, which, according to New Testament scholar Candida Moss, could be worded as "the power *leaked out* of him."[37] In other words, writes Morris, "Jesus' body becomes leaky, porous, and permeable—like that of a woman's." Again, we witness God cast in feminine terms, absorbing what we perceive as weakness into his own person, making it part of his ministry, his way of healing.

Taking in these images of God as a laboring woman and God as a porous, leaky woman, perhaps we can find in our deepest places of vulnerability and weakness something more—the presence of God. Perhaps there, as we face what was wielded to our harm, we can find the creative energy to offer it to God as something that can be used for our healing—and not just ours, but the world's.

Women's intimate bodily knowledge can be a way forward, an invitation for all of us to come home to our bodies, to care for our bodies and other bodies. Art historian Matthew Milliner writes that Mary, who bore God as an embryo in her body, was the first to practice what all Christians—men included—must follow. We are all called to receive God in our bodies, conceive God within us.[38] Women, as some theologians say, are the "pinnacle of creation." Our very porousness, connection, and embodiment may be exactly what God intended, exactly what this world needs. Perhaps if more leaders led out of a place of vulnerability—showing that we hurt too, admitting what we don't know and can't do—our world would look a bit more like

God's kingdom, where the last are first and weakness transmutes to strength (1 Corinthians 1:27; 2 Corinthians 12:9). Perhaps this is also why women, who know these places of vulnerability so well, are uniquely gifted for leadership.

The twelfth-century abbess Hildegard of Bingen understood that her body's vulnerability to illness also made her vulnerable to the Holy Spirit, writes Stephanie Paulsell: "She had what medieval medicine referred to as an 'airy temperament,' a bodily permeability that opened her both to recurring sickness and to God."[39] This might be said of all women, of all people whose bodies have been treated more as a liability than an asset in our current broken system. Our permeability—our vulnerability—if we let it, can open us up to God.

PART TWO

Becoming

WHOLE

6

VULNERABLE BODIES

I must confess that as a mother I don't have the most "maternal" reactions. Right after my second son turned two, that became obvious on the way home from a long road trip.

This son, nicknamed Weeds,[1] has always been more sensitive in his digestion. He was a colicky newborn, and for a few months in his first year he would wake up screaming every hour of the night. On a trip visiting family for Thanksgiving, we left behind his usual diet and let him eat a number of things he didn't usually—dairy, whole nuts, lots of cookies and dessert, and whatever restaurant food was convenient.

About halfway through our twelve-hour drive home, Weeds started crying, "Owie-owie-owie-owie." Since he didn't have many words to express himself, we had trouble figuring out what was bothering him. Was he tired of sitting in his car seat? Was he getting a sore throat? Did he have gas? In the passenger seat as my husband drove through a snowstorm, I turned around and tried to comfort him. But he continued to wail "owie," falling asleep intermittently and waking up again in distress.

Over the course of the next forty-eight hours or so, his pain got worse. He reverted to his newborn days, waking me up every hour of the night screaming. I finally took him to his pediatrician, where, after doing an x-ray, we discovered he was severely constipated. By this time the "owies" were coming out in a nonstop stream. After trying some over-the-counter laxatives, I ended up taking him to the ER late at night for an enema to get his bowels moving. That helped, but it wasn't the end. Weeds continued crying "owie-owie-owie," on and off for the next few days before his digestion gradually returned to normal.

My son's cries elicited that rush of anxiety, rapid heartbeat, and adrenaline that you would expect in any mother. But even at the beginning, as the "owies" dragged on in the car ride home from Thanksgiving, I felt the edge of a growing frustration, like a cold front moving in and icing over my heart. I was mad that Weeds was so sensitive and hurting and needy—and that I had to suffer for it. *At two years old,* I thought, *surely we should be over the night wakings. Surely he should be able to communicate what is the matter, instead of saying "owie" over and over.* I'm embarrassed to admit it, but there were times that week, as my nerves frayed and my anxiety mounted, that I burst out at Weeds to stop crying "owie" and couldn't find the resources within me to get up and comfort him yet again in the night. Thankfully, my husband was able to step in during those times when I couldn't muster up compassion for Weeds's "owies" anymore and just wanted to scream myself.

Unfortunately, I have a habit of getting frustrated when my kids (and Matt) are sick. I line up a battery of conventional and alternative treatments, try them all, and then stamp my foot in impatience when, after a couple days, the coughs and fevers linger and they still need so much round-the-clock attention. After Weeds's constipation incident, I tried to process some of these feelings with my husband.

How, I asked Matt, was he able to simply sit with Weeds in his pain without getting my fight-or-flight response? As we talked, I realized that my children's illnesses touch a raw nerve within me. I don't like seeing them so weak, so fragile, so hurting. I'm scared of their vulnerability. I don't like what it bodes for them, and for me, as their mother. I want to make the "owies" stop, because they remind me—over and over—that, often, I can't do anything more than wait for the illness to pass.

In the first part of this book, I've looked at some of the ways that we have been fragmented in body and soul. We fear our bodies—their imperfections, unpredictability, vulnerability, limits, and capacity to suffer—and so we distance ourselves. This fear tears us apart and we are left groping for a sense of identity, for wholeness. During chronic illness, when the raw edges of our human condition become the dull, aching center, we feel this fragmentation even more.

But what if the raw edges—these aspects of our physicality that we try to push out of our peripheral vision—are actually central to who we are as human beings? What if the vulnerability and limits we experience in illness tell a truer story about who we are than the invincibility and limit-pushing confidence we feel in good health? Or, at the very least, perhaps they tell an equally important story, one that gets missed in our rush to return to "normal."

How would embracing that story change how we live? How would that change who we are becoming? In the second half of this book, I dive into the aspects of our embodied existence that we shy away from, that we'd rather not identify with. Embracing them, I believe, is key to becoming whole.

"CULT OF NORMALCY"

I'm not alone in having a profoundly visceral and negative reaction to vulnerability. My feelings regarding my children's illnesses reflect what we value in middle-class North America. We recoil from neediness and dependence and prize autonomy and independence. A sick, hurting person relying on others is the opposite of the ideal American citizen who has pulled himself up by his bootstraps, pays his taxes, and contributes to the expansion of the gross domestic product. Nobody wants to be on the receiving end, and—though we may not admit it—we don't like to get too close to people who find themselves there repeatedly either. It feels embarrassing and uncomfortable, whether we're helping a frail older adult to the toilet or listening to a friend ask yet again for money to pay the rent. Why does vulnerability carry such social stigma?

Our society, writes theologian Thomas Reynolds, is built around the supposed unending growth of capitalism. The ultimate good, in this system, is production—making goods, offering services, investing and creating more wealth in a "virtuous cycle" of prosperity. We've come to value traits that make production possible—moving about freely, thinking rationally, and producing and purchasing goods in the market economy. Gradually, we've built a "cult of normalcy" around these ideals, Reynolds says—a yardstick that determines what kind of bodies measure up to our collective values, and what kind are inferior and peripheral.[2]

In this system, then, is it "normal" to require constant care and attention because of illness, disability, or old age? Increasingly, our society answers, "No." It's not "normal," because it doesn't fit into our grand project of economic growth. In North America, and increasingly in other parts of the world, we push those ill, disabled, or elderly bodies off to the side, into nursing homes and institutions where we can't see them, while we go about the "more important" work of production. This explains why traditional "women's work" is so undervalued—attending to the needs of vulnerable bodies doesn't add a penny to the company or national bottom line.

Recently, we've started pushing the expectations of productivity further out into the end of our lives. Scientists in the aging field are working on a range of treatments, from young blood infusions to removing old cells, that address the ailments of old age such as Alzheimer's, heart disease, and general decrepitude. While this goal of "compression of morbidity"— helping people age in a healthier way so they spend less years of their later life sick and dependent—is laudable, I wonder if it also creates an unrealistic expectation. We start to assume that it is "normal" to be healthy and live independently until the end of life. People who don't meet that expectation then see their bodies as "abnormal," and even their lives as less worth living.

Theologian Ephraim Radner suggested to me recently that the increasing acceptance of physician-assisted suicide might be the flip side to our society's preoccupation with "fixing" the vulnerabilities of aging and death. "We want to live longer. People are willing to spend the money to do that. Faced with the fact that they don't, faced with the fact that they're getting weaker, they can't even face the thought," he said. Radner notes that some European countries have expanded the criteria for "intolerable suffering" that could warrant physician-assisted suicide so that a few radically depressed teenagers have petitioned, and been allowed, to go through with it.[3]

Perhaps what makes our suffering so "intolerable" is that shame and embarrassment keep us from expressing it, from calling up a friend and saying, "I'm hurting. Can you help me?" In a wilderness of the body or emotions, we find ourselves alone, hemmed in by the walls of a self-imposed independence.

LONELINESS AND THE RISK OF PRESENCE

During my freshman year in college, I had grand expectations for making lifelong friends and living in an intense, bare-your-soul community. That did happen eventually, but the first few months were hard. I floundered as a transplant into white evangelical culture (I had not even heard the word *evangelical* until I arrived on campus). I missed jokes, misinterpreted social cues, and wondered if I would ever fit in, and if anyone cared. As fall faded into winter, I grew lonely and depressed. I had trouble falling asleep and concentrating on homework.

Ironically, at that juncture, I was assigned to present on the topic of loneliness for a required wellness class. In front of my well-groomed and bright-eyed peers, I choked out the words, "Loneliness can have serious effects on physical and mental health. It's important to combat social isolation to address loneliness." All the while, I couldn't bring myself to admit to my roommate, my RA, or my few friends that something was off inside. I worried that they would be repulsed by my neediness. I "compared my insides to others' outsides," something expressly forbidden in the book *10 Keys to Happier Living*,[4] and thought I was the only one who was insecure, the weakling who couldn't play in the big leagues. I missed my family. Some nights, I got up and wandered around campus at one a.m., crying and picking up pears from a tree near my dorm. I was abnormal.

By the end of freshman year, I did develop enough trust with some friends to ugly-cry in front of them and not pretend that everything was fine. By the next year, the depression was nonexistent. I had friends with whom I shared clothes, passed gas unabashedly, and held late-night conversations. I was not alone. But these relationships developed in fits and starts and required that I take the risk of being vulnerable, of showing my splotchy face and puffy eyes. I had to rely on other imperfect human beings instead of going it on my own. The latter would be admittedly safer, though probably not healthier.

If I were a college student now, I'd have many forms of technology available to let me take the route that felt safer. Current students utilize that technology freely. MIT scholar Sherry Turkle documents that today's young people have problems with in-person conversation. Growing up in an always-online culture, where you can escape any moment of boredom, loneliness, or awkward social tension by turning to your phone for distraction and affirmation, teens and college students don't know how to handle face-to-face interactions. They cringe at the meanderings, silences, and overlapping layers of verbal and nonverbal cues. One girl Turkle interviewed explains her anxieties this way:

> When we talk online, we talk about a whole bunch of stuff, but when I'm on the phone with a boy or in person, it's like "Ahh, mad awkward!" . . . Let's say you are both together face-to-face. Unless you come up with some kind of question or something, like if you say, "How was school?" or whatever, you've got nothing. And let's say he says, "Good," or "Fine." . . . You've still got nothing.[5]

Young people prefer to develop their relationships through social media or texting because it offers a "safer" route. You can rehearse and edit what you say. You can hide the furious blush spreading across your face. There are no uncomfortable silences, where people are simply present together, waiting for the others to respond or figuring out how to respond themselves. If there's a pause in a text or online thread, you assume that other people are busy managing their ten other digital interactions. If you don't know what to say next, you pretend that you are the busy one. Turkle's interviewees "make it clear that the back-and-forth of unrehearsed 'real-time' conversation is something that makes you 'unnecessarily' vulnerable."[6]

Families, too, have moved interactions online. Some prefer to argue via text, because "it makes things smoother," one teen says, and avoids facing those hot, messy emotions that always seem to bubble up. To these families, disagreements are now "more productive," with reduced risk that someone will say something they regret later.[7]

Yet, Turkle notes through one telling story, something is lost in the translation from face-to-face to online. Haley, a college student on break, often forgets to follow her family's house rule that if she stays out all night she has to text her parents. This results in predictable alarmed text messages from her mother, which Haley has gotten used to, and shrugs off. But one night, after Haley had stayed out all night without being in touch, her mom didn't send off her usual string of texts. Instead, she came down to breakfast the next morning to talk to her daughter in person. Haley says,

> I saw her face. My mom was almost crying. That can't be conveyed via text. She could be bawling. . . . If she sent a text, I wouldn't know. So in terms of sparking real reflection, there is something that is conveyed in emotions and facial expressions. . . . The way it made me feel didn't come from her words.[8]

I am struck again by how much we recoil from the body's vulnerability. In person, we can't hide that we are fragile, sensitive people who are deeply affected, often hurt, by the actions of those closest to us. Online, we can pretend we are safe, occupied with more important things. We can choose not to be present to our soft spots. We can hide our involuntary physical reactions. We can make like we aren't feeling disappointed, lonely, or scared.

But in person, the body doesn't lie. Tears well up and refuse to stay contained. Lips twitch downward into a grimace. Skin turns pink and mottled. We can see our bodies as liabilities, revealing those tender parts that we prefer to keep hidden. Or we can see them as God-given points of connection that tell the true story of who we are, even when we can't put words to it. Even as we fear the risks of human connection, our bodies reach out for it, soliciting empathy and sending SOS signals in the hopes that they will reach another human being and bring them back to us, bringing us together.

NO LONGER EXCEPTIONAL

It's one thing to risk vulnerability with family and friends, those we know and trust. It's another to do so with strangers. Building walls to protect "our people" seems to be a natural human response to any kind of perceived threat. As a mother, invisible threats to my children's health—like toxins and germs—pushed me toward trying to create "pure" environments for them, as if by my own grit I could blow a magic bubble around their delicate little bodies, keeping all the monsters outside. In 2019, the president of the United States was pushing relentlessly to build a wall along our southern border, keeping out "illegal aliens" with the real and imagined dangers they pose. During the Ebola crisis of 2013 to 2014 in Liberia and surrounding countries, medical workers who went overseas to help were not lauded as heroes, but as foolish risk-takers who might bring the virus back home. During the COVID-19 pandemic, we learned how porous our boundaries are. Travel bans and border closings couldn't keep the virus out.

When we come against danger, our first instinct is to externalize the threat—to find a scapegoat. We cast blame on those who are outside our group, whether undocumented immigrants or Africans with unsanitary burial practices or Asians. Like early American settlers, we take on a frontier mentality, imagining our bodies as isolated homesteads. "The health of the homestead next to ours does not affect us, this thinking suggests, so long as ours is well tended," Eula Biss writes.[9] This mentality makes the threats seem more manageable, because it gives us a way to control them. We want to believe we can pull ourselves above the crowd, that the problems that affect "them" are not relevant to us, because we are, somehow, exceptional.

Growing up as a 1.5-generation immigrant in the United States, I absorbed my fair share of this American myth that told me I could do anything I wanted if I tried hard enough.[10] My status as a member of several marginalized groups—a female, an ethnic minority, with undocumented parents—could have brought me to an earlier reckoning with the structures that keep this myth from becoming a reality for many. But my parents were relatively successful, despite our setbacks, and bought into the myth themselves. In fact, being a child of upwardly mobile immigrants amplified my feeling that I was exceptional. *Here we are,* I thought, *hustling to run a Chinese restaurant, saving, buying a house without debt, and lifting ourselves above all these folks stuck in their small-town Texas ruts.*

They were born here; they will stay here. But I'm going to move on and get out of here. I'm better than these people.

I'm wiser now. I know about systemic injustice, baked-in racism, generational poverty, and the unique problems of rural working-class America. But in small ways, even today, I live out the idea that I am above the rules that everyone else must follow, because I am more clever, resourceful, and informed. In traffic jams, for example, I refuse to believe I will be late and instead leave the expressway for small roads, putting distance between me and the rest of the honking, impatient mass of stuck humanity.

In the aftermath of the 2008 financial crisis, as our peers struggled to find jobs and make ends meet, my husband and I managed to do pretty well. We paid off our loans, put away some money, and got into the real-estate market at its lowest point. This was purely a matter of being in the right place at the right time. We also had parents who passed on their real-estate acumen and lent us part of the down payment. But part of me still wants to believe that we are somehow hacking it better than everyone else. Maybe home foreclosures and working at Starbucks for years is only something that happens to other people, not us.

Disaster is one of the surest paths to disabusing ourselves of the illusion that we can, by sheer force of will, insulate ourselves from harm. For me, these lessons have come through chronic pain, along with my children's many health scares.

The scales fell off my eyes one afternoon, early on in my own pain, as I sat with my foot propped up in our newlywed shoebox apartment. Matt was at work, and without anyone to shake me out of the funk, I repeatedly hit replay on the "Why me?" monologue streaming in my head. At this point, I was still grasping for a reason, assuming (unconsciously) that bad things didn't just *happen*, at least not to me. Then, still asking why, my imagination drifted toward the bad things that happen to other people—the couple at church with their stillborn child, the families fleeing bombs in Afghanistan, the handful of people I knew who had cancer. The sudden realization felt like free-falling on the Tower of Terror ride at Disney: actually, I was no different from all these people. They were taking their very best whack at life, and still death, war, and disease struck. All their best efforts didn't protect them. They were naked and exposed in the face of tragedy. And so was I. I was no better.

It was terrifying.

"[God] makes his sun rise on the evil and on the good, and sends rain on the righteous and on the unrighteous," Jesus said (Matthew 5:45). He also asked, regarding the eighteen who were killed in the fall of the tower of Siloam, "Do you think that they were worse offenders than all the others living in Jerusalem?" (Luke 13:4-5). The answer is no. Bad things happen to the best of us. Realizing I was as vulnerable as the next person was part of what plunged me into depression in my early years of chronic pain. I felt, now, that in addition to asking why to my own suffering I had to ask for everyone else as well. And, of course, there are no easy answers.

But it's difficult to live in such a state. Even as we are constantly reminded of our fragility, we humans manage to spend many of our waking hours in denial, acting as if we will live forever, shielding our eyes from the shadows lurking in the corners.

How else can we live with our vulnerability, besides ignoring it and posturing invincibility, being existentially paralyzed by it, or pretending like it's outside of ourselves and walling ourselves off from danger? Here is where we need the gospel.

TRANSFORMING VULNERABILITY

Philippians 2:5-8 has always been one of my favorite passages of Scripture:

> Let the same mind be in you that was in Christ Jesus,
>> who, though he was in the form of God,
>>> did not regard equality with God
>>> as something to be exploited,
>> but emptied himself,
>>> taking the form of a slave,
>>> being born in human likeness.
> And being found in human form,
>> he humbled himself
>> and became obedient to the point of death—
>> even death on a cross.

I love its upside-down nature. Jesus Christ may be the one truly exceptional human being, in that he joins both human and divine in an inextricable whole. But instead of playing his privilege card to get himself out of the massive traffic pile-on that is our human condition, he stays. Even more, he bends lower, all the way down to the deepest pit that we could dig for ourselves—death. He identifies himself completely with our vulnerability, taking it into his own nature. He lets himself be utterly destroyed by the consequences. Where our impulse is to escape, to self-protect, to rise above, Jesus chooses to surrender, to give himself up, to descend.

The story, of course, doesn't end with Jesus' death, but continues with his resurrection. He pushes past death and tells us, from the other side, "Do not be afraid" (Matthew 28:10). *You think you will lose your life by surrendering to vulnerability, but it is not complete annihilation. It is transformation.* He says to followers in John 12:24, "Unless a grain of wheat falls into the earth and dies, it remains just a single grain; but if it dies, it bears much fruit." In his life, death, and resurrection, Jesus shows us a new way to live. When we press into those places of deep pain and loss with him, where it feels like all the life is being squeezed out, we find not a permanent grave, but a tunnel opening up to a different kingdom. Here, the last are first, weakness is strength, and servants become rulers. Sharing our resources results in their multiplication, and depending on others reinforces, rather than diminishes, our dignity.

At Jesus' ascension, he passes on his mission to his followers. Then at Pentecost, he imbues us with his Spirit. The church becomes his physical presence on earth, his very body. He has no other way to be here in flesh and blood, except through our bodies. This, too, says Lauren Winner, is an act of vulnerability: "The calling of the church—the naming of a collection of human beings as God's own body—makes God vulnerable to our continued failings, our continued rejections, our continued refusals to be God's body."[11] In other words, God now depends on us.

In Winner's discussion of God as a laboring woman from Isaiah 42, we observe that, though God is the one birthing a new creation, we are God's midwives, doulas, assistants. He has made us his partners. For example, Winner notes that in the opening verses of that chapter, listeners are urged to "sing to the LORD a new song" (v. 10). This parallels the ways singing and music have helped women through labor both in ancient societies and today. It suggests "a sort of Mobius strip of redemption," Winner reflects, "in which God is redeeming, God is suffering the pains of redemption, and, as we are being redeemed, the new song we sing helps—helps God breathe, helps God relax, helps God feel less pain, helps God deliver."[12]

Disability advocate Judith Snow goes even further with the idea of God's dependence, offering the image of God as a paraplegic. As a paraplegic doesn't have use of their limbs and thus relies on personal assistants, so God relies on us.[13] The image is startling, like the picture of God as a laboring woman. It points to how God raises up those aspects of our human experience that some deem inferior, undignified, and repulsive—like our neediness—and transforms them into sources of power and grace. This is what he did in the crucifixion and resurrection. It is what he does now in our own unique struggles, whether with chronic illness, sick children, or everyday bodily discomforts.

WHERE GOD MEETS US

My maternal grandmother, whom I called "Waipo," died recently, at the age of eighty-nine. She was eating a meal when suddenly she could no longer lift up the chopsticks to her mouth and fell into a coma. Her heart stopped beating a couple days later.

Waipo raised seven children in Mao-era China, when food shortages and social upheaval were commonplace. She survived the drowning of her first husband (my biological grandfather) when my mother was nine years old. In her last couple decades, Waipo didn't maintain her own home, but spread her days and things between children, staying with one child for a few months, then another. It wasn't always harmonious, and, toward the end, as Waipo grew more needy and childlike, my aunts and uncles felt the burden of care more acutely, with some annoyance.

During Waipo's last days and passing, though, my family rose to the occasion. They worried about leaving her alone in the ICU while she was in a coma, not wanting her to die cold and unaccompanied. After her death, my aunts bathed and dressed her body. In her casket, they covered her with seven blankets, symbolizing her seven children. Her funeral display was a riot of plates piled with fruit, burning incense, hanging lanterns, and Chinese calligraphy, all celebrating the bonds of love and interdependence Waipo wove throughout her life.

My family's respect for Waipo during her most profound moment of vulnerability—death—models for me the ways we are called to respond to the vulnerabilities in ourselves and others. We show up. We stay present.

There are other notable examples: Mother Teresa's homes for the dying in Calcutta; the L'Arche communities; death accompaniment programs, where volunteers take turns sitting beside dying people without next of kin in hospitals or nursing homes. We see, in these instances, how weakness calls out in us our deepest, most noble human instinct—to see in the face of every person the image of God, and then, to give each person the attention and care worthy of that image, regardless of ability, social standing, or productivity.

In these models, we see that when we are stripped naked of the many layers of protection we've built around ourselves, such as wealth, status, intellect, health—the things we grasp onto to reassure ourselves that we will be okay—we come closest to God. We stand before him and others needy and dependent, knowing in our flesh and bones the truth that we came into the world with nothing and we leave with nothing. Each of us is simply a human being with nothing more to offer than ourselves. This is a sacred place where God meets us. When we have nothing to give, we are enough. We are loved. We are holy. Simply because we are God's own.

When we give and receive in these moments, we are joined to others in webs of mutual interdependence. Sometimes we give more; sometimes we receive more. Sometimes we think we are simply meeting another's needs, but actually we are being transformed ourselves in the process. We belong to each other. If we can acknowledge these ties, to those close and far, we are on our way to becoming truly human. Self-sustaining independence is an illusion whose pursuit only leaves us in fragments. Vulnerability—acknowledging our deficits and relying on others to meet us in those deficits—is the only way to true selfhood, to wholeness.

Theologian William Placher illustrates this with the analogy of a basketball team. If players are concerned with their personal performance in comparison to others, trying to be the MVP by making the most shots and standing out, then they will never play to their potential. But if they lose themselves in the game and give their all to winning as a team, then these players actually end up becoming the best players, involved in a kind of "self-forgetfulness that paradoxically made them the best players, as individuals, that they have ever been." He continues, "Acknowledging my limits, making myself vulnerable in full relation to an other is the only way I can become fully myself. Such loss of self-independence in relation does not threaten individual identity but precisely creates it."[14]

Theologian Joyce Ann Mercer has also reflected on vulnerability and interdependence in helpful ways. What do older adults have to offer, she asks, when they can't work and can't take care of themselves? Do they have a calling? She believes they do, and points us toward an understanding of calling that goes beyond what we normally imagine it to be—what we *do* and how we are *useful*—to a "relational ecology."[15] "Absent of the features that play such a critical role in the preceding years of middle and even late adulthood," she explains, "we instead find older adult vocation particularly emphasizing *who* we are as creatures of God, *how* we are in relationship (with God, with others), and *what* capacities we evoke in others, rather than what we produce or accomplish." Older adults, as care receivers, evoke in others the "practices, habits, and dispositions of faithful people"—that is, people who honor the image of God in others. Like children, the way older adults experience time, not as something to be spent and managed but as "a space of grace where relationships unfold," invites their caregivers to slow down and be present.[16]

In addition, because of their declining health, older adults' bodies come to the forefront and remind us of our creaturehood. As Mercer says:

> Older adulthood's amplified awareness of bodies, their limits and possibilities, underscores God's creation of human beings for vocation as the very embodied creatures we are, and not in spite of our bodies. Even when aging bodies seem to offer more hindrances than aid to our participation in God's reconciling love, in this life we do not have the option for *ad extra* vocation, the living out of God's calling beyond the body.

Bodies matter in God's call and how we respond, Mercer stresses.[17]

When my children are sick or when I am in pain, I'd much rather respond to God's call in a way that transcends the body. In these instances, when I have been up multiple times in the night and can barely keep my eyes open to write down thoughts on a page, the body's weaknesses seem like an unnecessary liability; they keep me from the work I want to do. I take Weeds's "owies" as a nuisance, a distraction from the real task at hand.

But then, by God's grace, I occasionally experience little pockets of a deeper reality. As Weeds quiets down and sucks his thumb, using his other hand to trace the edge of my fingernails over and over (one of those quirky self-soothing tools that all babies develop), I sink into a lull where nothing else matters but being with him, our bodies touching, knowing that my physical presence is a comfort to him, and his to me. He needs me, and I need him. And that is okay. It is good. The fact that I can meet him in his pain and vulnerability is what makes me human. It also teaches him what being human is all about. Weeds is learning, I hope, that it is okay to express his pain to others, okay to ask for help. He is practicing how to relate to God and others in the inevitable suffering he will experience throughout his life.

SHOWING UP

"To exist," writes theologian Norman Wirzba, "is necessarily to be rooted and entangled within places with a multitude of (seen and unseen) others. Our essential work is not liberation from places or from others. It is, rather, to learn the art of hospitality, which welcomes, nurtures, and releases others into the fullness of their lives, so that our presence contributes to the healing and flourishing of all."[18]

Wirzba highlights what is required for healing—presence and hospitality. They are two sides of the same coin. If we can show up fully as the mixed-up bundles of needs, questions, and gifts that we are ourselves, we can then receive others fully as their own mixed-up bundles of needs, questions, and gifts. To be vulnerable and live into wholeness, we practice the art of simply showing up.

It sounds basic, but it requires courage. It required me to hold on to my little boy writhing in pain, even when I couldn't do anything to stop it. It requires those of us who are sick and hurting to let others in on how we really feel, to tell them what we need. We often worry that our needs will be a burden, making others feel obligated. But there is a way to express our vulnerability that can be a gift to ourselves and others.

Grace once started having a migraine in the middle of giving a presentation for class. She had to ask the professor to turn the lights down in order to compose herself, while her classmates looked on. She finished the presentation, but slurred and tripped over her words, she was so frazzled. "It felt so humiliating, being stripped of words and any sense of clarity of thought or speech. . . . But after I got over it and reflected on it, it reminded me that I'm not what I produce and not what I perform," she said. I imagine that when Grace gave herself permission to pause and name her needs, others in the room also received permission to do the same themselves. She became part of creating a culture of vulnerability.

Because we often need so much when we are sick and hurting—whether it's different foods, access to seats or bathrooms at inconvenient times, dim lights, or leaving early from social gatherings—it can be easier to simply stay home. Pain and illness are socially isolating because we don't know how to be sick and hurting in front of others. Like our young people on their devices, we don't know how to bring our bodies to the table.

After the onset of Kimberly's fibromyalgia, she spent years avoiding certain group situations because she didn't know if she would be able to get what she needed among others with different needs and expectations. She also didn't want to be perceived as "high maintenance." Recently she took a risk and joined three other women for a conference that involved three nights away from home.

"I was terrified," she said. She really needed to sleep in a room by herself, so when someone brought it up, she put that need on the table, feeling her heart racing as she did so. On the drive, she had to stop by a store to get foods she could eat, given her dietary restrictions. As the conference wrapped up on the first night, Kimberly was in a lot of pain and was done for the day. She wanted to respect that her companions still wanted to stay and socialize, so she sat down and put her head on the table, off to the side away from the hubbub. Throughout the trip, Kimberly practiced being present and tending to her body's needs even as she recognized the needs and desires of others in her group.

By the end of the conference, on the car ride home, something had changed for her. Kimberly choked up when she told the other women, "I want to thank you guys for letting me be where I'm at. I realize I have been very socially hidden or held back because I'm so scared of needing so much when I'm in a social situation." The others affirmed her. They appreciated that she didn't say, "Take me home" on the first night. But they were also glad she let them know she needed to sleep in a room by herself. Kimberly and her companions were able to work out vulnerability and healthy boundaries in real time, face to face.

Kimberly learned to name her needs, without dismissing others' needs. She gave others a chance to meet her needs and be with her, rather than get angry or withdraw. "That was me fully showing up," she said. "I wasn't lacking, because I required all those things. In fact, I felt more whole."

7

OUR HUMAN LIMITS

*O*ne winter I had exactly two working limbs—a left hand and a right foot.

I had started graduate classes at the University of Chicago, which meant getting from our apartment in Oak Park, the closest suburb west of Chicago, to the campus in Hyde Park on the city's south side. The commute was a one-and-a-half-hour ride along the entire length of the Green Line, a short bus stint across Washington Park, and lots of walking and standing in between, not to mention crossing campus multiple times for classes. My ankle couldn't handle all of that walking (I could barely limp down the block), so my husband and I found an ingenious solution—transport by scooter.

This was not your typical flimsy kid's toy. It was a Xootr—made especially for adults with a birchwood deck wide as a skateboard and 180-millimeter polyurethane wheels with aluminum hubs. The ride was *smooth*—and really fun. I could keep my left foot planted on the deck, minimizing the repetitive motions that caused pain, while letting my right foot do the work. Riding the short stretch from the train to our apartment on an empty, tree-lined street, I was able to pick up enough speed for the wind to make my clothes flap, and I relished again the feeling of using my body to get places. I had missed that feeling.

Once winter hit, though, some unknown combination of factors made my pain flare up, to the point that even standing on the scooter was uncomfortable. I needed to give my ankle a complete rest, but I still had classes to attend and a part-time job in downtown Chicago. I had also started doing thesis research in Chinatown, which meant more stairs and scooting and time up and about. Reluctantly, I pulled out a pair of garage-sale crutches that I had used the summer before. *What would draw less attention,* I thought to myself, *scooting around on an overgrown child's toy or using crutches?* Neither. I sighed. Hopefully a couple days off the ankle would be enough to calm it down.

It turned out that all that crutching was more than my wrists could handle. The next day, my usually bony right wrist swelled thick and balloon-like. Moving my fingers caused hot pain. Now, I couldn't crutch or walk. Nor could I type notes in class or stuff envelopes for my job. In our tiny rented space above a garage, I squinted from worry and tears, trying to read about the atrophy and adaptation of China's Communist Party for one of my classes while soaking my wrist in a warm Epsom salt bath.

Somehow I muddled my way through the next few weeks. I quit my part-time job, skipped a few days of classes, and cobbled together a bizarre shorthand to type one-handed notes during lectures. My wrist returned to its usual size and my ankle calmed down enough to go back to scooting, but the entire episode heightened my anxiety.

Not long after, Matt and I met a friend for dinner in Chinatown after I finished some research. Over Mapo tofu and stir-fried Chinese broccoli, my ankle started to throb more than usual. *Uh-oh,* I thought, *not this again.* I kept the alarming thoughts at bay until we got on the train to go home. The fluorescent glare of lights and the feeling of zooming along in the darkness late at night quickened my despairing spiral of thoughts. Each ding-dong of a train stop marked a tightening in the viselike grip of anxiety. Soon, everything crystallized into one driving need—*I must go to the emergency room now. I must get this ankle taken care of. It can't get worse or I'll be back to two working limbs again, maybe one, maybe none! I can't handle this anymore. They'll have something at the hospital to fix me.*

Matt always gets the brunt of my unfiltered, unchecked anxiety (isn't that what spouses are for?). Barreling along the rickety tracks, I declared to him my plans.

"You're being irrational," he whispered. "We don't need to go to the hospital at midnight for your ankle. It's already been hurting for two years. You've seen so many doctors and done so many treatments. What makes you think that going to the ER now is going to be any different? It can wait till morning."

"You're ignoring my pain," I whispered back fiercely, nearly in tears. "You don't know what this feels like!" We went back and forth like this until the Oak Park exit, when he grabbed the bag of leftovers and huffed off the train without waiting for me. I followed him mournfully, down the platform stairs and across the street, watching the distance between us increase.

When I turned the corner to catch sight of him again, I saw him snap. He threw the bag of leftovers onto the sidewalk, as if slamming a basketball to make it bounce high, and tofu and broccoli bits exploded out. Then he kicked the bag for good measure.

I winced, and felt my own heart harden. I wouldn't go home. I would sit outside in the bitter cold on an empty planter and let him stew until he felt bad, which I knew he would eventually. After about twenty minutes, though, my fingers started going numb, and I relented. I went inside and found him with his head in his hands. "I'm so sorry," he mumbled. I didn't go to the ER that night.

LIMITS: NEUTRAL, UNSURPRISING, AND INTRINSIC TO OUR HUMANITY

We laugh ruefully about "the Chinese food incident" now. When I brought it up recently, Matt shared his take: "I was really tired. I didn't want to start another ordeal at the hospital and be there for hours and have to work the next morning. I was trying to balance my needs with yours—I guess that's all of marriage—and I'm probably not as selfless as some people." I appreciated his honest grappling with the balance. Partners and friends of people with chronic conditions can't be expected to put their needs second all the time. They have limits too.

Looking back, it's tragically comical—how angry my husband got, how desperate I was to be fixed. How delighted some neighborhood dog must have been out on a walk the next morning. Yet the core desire I felt was quite serious. I wanted a quick fix. I wanted to overcome my body's failures and limits. I thought I could find a solution through medicine and technology.

That same desire drives many of our modern endeavors. Entire industries, such as technology or anti-aging, aim to help us achieve more, live longer, and go faster and farther than we have in the past. There are people today who live as if death is optional, who treat the frailties of our bodies as technical glitches with equally technical solutions—treatable, with enough time and money. Our finite, embodied existence is seen as a flaw. And, we reason, if pushing the limits is good, then limits must be bad. We have made it normal to raise the bar higher and higher—think about the never-ending quest to grow the economy and have a continually rising GDP. It is abnormal to stay put, to say, "This is as far as we can go."

Yet, what could be more normal than having limits? If having a body is an undeniable part of being human, and if bodies are, by nature, limited, then being human means having limits. These limits are not inherently bad or good. They just *are*. Deborah Beth Creamer, in *Disability and Christian Theology*, calls limits a neutral, unsurprising part of being human.[1]

The nature of being a particular human being is a case in point. I am Liuan Chen Huska, a woman who was born to Yimin and Fusheng in the People's Republic of China and who grew up in the United States of America. If I am Liuan, I can't be Maria. If I am a woman, I can't be a man (leaving transgender discussions aside). I am Chinese American, and not Russian or Togolese. I can't pick new biological parents or generate new DNA for myself (though perhaps this will be possible sometime in the near future). My specific, human identity limits my ability to be any number of other specific, human identities. This is not bad. It simply is the way things are. I carry these neutral markers on my body, though society can interpret them in positive and negative ways. My body serves as a boundary line. I am Liuan, up to the edges of my skin. Then I stop, and the rest of the world, including other people, begins.

Paradoxically, our bodies both limit and connect. I can't get out of my body to experience what another person is thinking and feeling, and they can't get into mine. But without my body, I would have no way of reaching out to other human beings. I wouldn't be able to sit on a chair and eat granola for breakfast with my little boys, or hug Gloria in church while her perfume rubs off on me, or even use my fingers and eyes to type out these words. And my body is, in fact, the only way I can meet with God—in the minutiae of my daily living. I can't fly away into the sky on the wings of the spirit and become sanctified there. God meets me here, in this crumbly Communion bread and "two-buck Chuck" Trader Joe's wine, here in my near-sighted eyes and winter-chapped skin. In the particular, we encounter the holy.

God, in the incarnation of Jesus, lived out this paradox of bodily limitation and connection. He became human, because he knew that to make his love accessible to us earth-bound creatures, he would have to show it to us in very concrete ways—eating fish by the lake, washing feet, rubbing blind eyes with saliva and dirt, pouring out water and blood on a cross. He became a body and voluntarily assumed all the limits and vulnerabilities that come with it. He became *just like us.*

This means that he didn't have access to a divine credit card, theologian Cherith Fee Nordling says. Everything he did, from walking on water to feeding thousands, was done out of the partial unknowing that all of us operate with. The only difference is that Jesus maintained perfect obedience to his Father and ongoing connection to the Holy Spirit within him, who empowered all his "superhuman" acts. Nordling thus reads the feeding of the five thousand this way: Before it happened, Jesus didn't think, *Okay, now it's time to do a miracle.* He didn't know beforehand all that his Father would do through him. In that moment, as he raised the bread and fish in thanksgiving, he submitted himself to whatever God intended, and let the Spirit's power flow. That power, channeled through human hands, multiplied meager portions to feed a crowd.[2]

Jesus wasn't just God pretending to be human. He *was*, and *is still,* human. And it is precisely *through* Jesus' humanity, *because* he had a body, along with all the limits that bodies entail, that he was able to get through to us, to bridge the distance between God and people, to join the human and the divine. Jesus' bounded, human body connects us with God.

LIMITS IN THE RESURRECTION

Despite all we know about Jesus, we still try to escape our earthly groundings. We have found many ways to split body and spirit, assuming that physical limits are only temporary and that Jesus came to free us from these entrapments so that we can be whole in eternity. Take this quote by Marva Dawn, for example: "Let us, then, concentrate not on the manner in which our diminished bodies are breaking down, but on the splendors of the limitless life that we shall enjoy eventually."[3] I don't take issue with her anticipation of the life to come (and, in general, I think she has many wise things to say), but I wonder if "limitless" is the most helpful way to describe life in our resurrected bodies. It may be true that some of the limits we endure now—aging, death, the ravages of disease—will not continue into eternity (thanks be to God). And Jesus' own acts in the forty days he was on earth after his resurrection suggest that our bodies won't operate entirely according to the same physical laws that govern now. He entered the disciples' room despite locked doors and disappeared from view right after breaking bread with the disciples walking to Emmaus.

But to hint that our life will be limitless is to say in a roundabout way that we won't have bodies. Will we be in all places at once? Will we see and know everything? These attributes, which we normally attribute to God the Father, imply the bodiless life of a spirit-being, not the life of a human being who lives within skin at a particular place and time. It doesn't seem to fit the life of the resurrected Jesus, either, who ate fish on a lake and hugged his friends and, after his ascension, was "not there" anymore.

Perhaps there is one way in which Dawn's idea of a "limitless life" is accurate. As Jesus ascended into heaven, he commanded his disciples to stay in Jerusalem until they received the gift of the Holy Spirit. He knew that his people would not be able to continue his work on earth on their own. They needed power beyond themselves, power that transcended their human limits. They needed the Holy Spirit. This Spirit, whom each believer receives, binds disparate individuals into one body, a mystical body that is more than the sum of its parts and transcends time and space. Because the Spirit dwells in each of us who belongs to Jesus, we can say that we participate in a limitless life, even now, because we are connected to the larger body of Christ and plugged into a bottomless source of love and power. But this is not because we have—or will—shed our bodies. It is because we are part of a Body bigger than our selves.

The most straightforward interpretation of "limitless," however, is still problematic. Conceiving of the resurrected life as limitless shines a negative light on all limits and makes transcending bodily limits something to strive for now.

WHEN WE PUSH THE LIMITS

After college, I landed my first job at a Christian nonprofit. A handful of other coworkers and I worked doggedly under a visionary but impractical director to organize one week in June full of seminars, workshops, mentorships, networking dinners, concerts, book sales, focus groups, and more for over four hundred church leaders. As the week approached, eight-hour days stretched into nine, ten, or more. The director operated with a heartfelt burden for the conference attendees, who lived in countries with few resources and networks to support their work.

While I found the mission deeply meaningful, on a day-to-day basis this burden translated to me and my coworkers as a constant pressure to work harder and longer. This was a ministry, and people depended on us. We couldn't stop, or even scale back, because that would be shortchanging all these people who needed us, skimping on God's work. The director had no sense of human limits.

A few days before the conference, my coworkers and I lugged suitcases of materials onto an overseas plane ride and hit the ground running upon arrival, shrugging off jet lag and mounting fatigue. We scrambled to solve logistical emergencies, sometimes fueled by another idea from the director that *had* to be implemented; no opportunities were wasted as long as there were willing workers. I spent very few hours in my hotel room and many hours in the conference hallways, running from here to there, worrying that something might not go off as planned. On one of the last nights, after a team meeting with the director where we were patted on the back for a job well done, one of my coworkers and I collapsed into each other's arms and cried.

My husband and I spent the next two weeks traveling. At our first destination, a Tuscan villa surrounded by olive trees, I sat in a swing and stared out at the distant hills. I couldn't do anything else. Matt told me later that I acted strangely on that trip, though in the moment I don't remember doing so. I sometimes didn't finish sentences or didn't answer questions. I cried over trivial things. Once, we got lost in the historic inner city of Seville. He drove while I was supposed to help him navigate. I ended up crying helplessly while he took the GPS out of my hands and parked the car. Then I followed him out, gazing blankly at the beautiful surroundings while he led us through the maze of cobblestone paths until we finally found our hostel, where I fell into the bed and cried some more.

I learned through this experience that when we push the override button one too many times, eventually our bodies say "no." This "no" comes in many forms—headaches, body aches, tightness in the chest, hormonal imbalances, rashes, stomach cramps, etc. After that conference, my body responded to my overrides of the preceding weeks with thick, cottony brain fog and easily triggered tears. All of these physical, mental, and emotional responses are the body's way of making us slow down and pay attention, of reminding us that we are, indeed, humans who need to eat, sleep, and rest. In some cases, our bodies put on the brakes for a short time but then allow us to return to living at "normal" speed. In other cases, the symptoms drag on, evading quick fixes, and we have to come to terms with what might be a chronic illness.[4]

In the United States, nearly half of the population lives with a condition that would be classified as a chronic illness—including conditions like heart disease and diabetes—and the percentage is growing.[5] Worldwide, the rate of autoimmune disorders, a subset of chronic illness, is also increasing.[6] The numbers are rising partly because we live longer than past generations. The risk of getting some diseases (like cancer and heart disease) compounds with age. Genetics, lifestyle (like diets high in processed foods and lack of physical activity), and environmental exposures also factor in.

I wonder if the rise in chronic illnesses in our time might be interpreted as our bodies' ongoing protests, a way of pulling out all the stops to say that something is terribly, terribly wrong about how we live today. Some of it might be traced to individual hubris, like that feeling I sometimes have that I can't stop because the show can't go on without me. More fault, though, lies in our collective drive to push past our limits.

We human beings, Americans in particular, have elevated unfettered economic growth above listening to our bodies and the bodies of the most vulnerable in our midst—including the poor, children, animals, and the sacred body of the earth. We pump harmful chemicals into our air and water in the name of being business-friendly and feed nutrient-poor processed foods to our kids because it's cheap and sells the best. We've set up a rat race of making money and buying things, beating our bodies up to get ahead and produce more, with little idea to what end. Even the most idealistic and disciplined among us have a hard time not falling into that race at some point.

We haven't honored our bodies or their limits, and, unsurprisingly, our bodies are saying "no."

A NARROW CHANNEL

One of my favorite college professors loved to throw around the phrase "five-thousand-channel universe" to critique the endless, mind-numbing, and often insignificant choices that we are offered each day in our click-bait, Instagrammable society. The phrase sticks with me as I think about the limits imposed on us by our bodies, whether we are healthy or sick. The very nature of our bodies—that we get sick, that we all die, that we need sleep, that we can't fly—undermines our collective illusion of unfettered economic growth and individualism.

However, a five-thousand-channel universe is a far cry from the simple things we ask out of life, things that don't seem to push the boundaries that much. Was it too much for me to ask to walk around the block without pain? Or for a mother with rheumatoid arthritis to hope she can decorate the Christmas tree with her kids? Sick people aren't looking for five thousand channels; we are simply praying for one option, or maybe a couple, for a decent life. It often seems, instead, that all channels are blocked. Pain, endless afternoons in doctors' waiting rooms, and tormented nights cloud the vision and obscure the way forward. Can our spirit, ambitions, and zest for life really be squeezed through a pinhole?

In one of the worst points of my pain and depression—it was February 2011—a massive snowstorm hit the Chicago area. For once, these hearty Midwesterners I lived among called a snow day. No school, no work, no Metra trains, no leaving the house. The exception was my husband, who dove through the four-foot snowdrifts and got to his office building, one block away from our apartment. Alone in our shoebox apartment, I emailed some of my friends and asked them to join me in prayer and fasting. I was turning the snow day into my own God-I'm-Banging-on-Your-Door-So-You'd-Better-Answer Day.

I felt trapped in a months-long cycle of trying to get better. I was fed up with trying doctors and treatments, but not doing anything also seemed unthinkable, equivalent to accepting that this pain would be here for a long time, maybe for the rest of my life. I couldn't handle the thought of that, emotionally. I was twenty-two. I wanted to be out trekking the Swiss Alps, not crutching down Main Street in Wheaton, Illinois. Life was not supposed to be this way.

I spent a lot of that day lying on a green yoga mat, crying, journaling, prayer-dancing. I stared at the ceiling more often than not. What I wanted was for God to show me some clear direction forward. I wanted to know that whatever next step I took was the right path, that I was not moving in circles. I wanted reassurance that I would get better, even if it took a while. I wanted to feel that God was with me. That he was *doing something* for me.

I didn't receive what I was hoping for that day. I didn't see a fork in the road clearly lit. I received no words or images that might be taken as a clue for what to do next. What I sensed from God was this: *You can still be part of my kingdom, whatever happens next.* It was simply an affirmation of meaning and purpose in the midst of limits that I wanted so badly to escape. Having that as the conclusion of my snow-pray day was frustrating. I didn't find a way out of the pain and confusion. I was still practically in the same place physically, emotionally, and spiritually. But I realized I had a choice about whether or not to trust that God could make something out of what seemed like not much to work with. At least not much that I wanted to work with.

Nothing dramatic happened afterward. The most concrete response I could muster was to bring fresh fruit with me to my part-time job in downtown Chicago to give to the panhandlers and homeless people who lined the busy streets. (I always felt bad passing them but didn't feel comfortable giving money.) I kept drifting from day to day in a fog of tears and griping at God. But at least I did keep going. It would take a long while for me to accept that I would never go back to the old normal.

The one additional resource I had, though, was this invitation from God. *Do you trust that I can squeeze the abundant life*

I want to give you through this pinhole, this eye of the needle, this (to you) absurdly narrow channel? Will you open your eyes and look around? I am the river, deep and untamable. Will you dive in? Or will you crouch at the rocky edge, clutching all you can't let go of? I could take or leave this invitation. Some days I took it. Some days I left it.

I admire the people who have taken up this invitation to life, to creativity, to strike rocks with sticks in the desert and find water gushing forth—or at least taken it up more often than I have. There is Laura, an artist and teacher who has created art in conversation with the limits imposed on her by hearing loss due to a condition called cholesteatoma. Laura underwent eleven surgeries in ten years, a little over half of them attempts to restore some of her hearing. She has mourned the time she spent in her twenties in doctors' waiting rooms instead of engaged in meaningful relationships. Yet, out of the tension between what she wants to do and what she has to do to tend to her body, she has created something.

Laura's master's thesis focused on visualizing the activity of beehives, a project inspired by her own hearing loss and her desire to find other ways to experience sound. Also, because she spent so much time in waiting rooms, Laura ended up making some very small pieces of art—portable enough to take to and from doctors' offices. She completed a residency at an artists' guild where she delved deeper into the ideas of the waiting room as studio as well as the use of art in the medical and hospital contexts. These projects all came out of Laura's willingness to engage with the frustration of having limits, rather than ignore or escape them.

Pat has also navigated the narrow channel life has given her with grace and imagination. She has lived with various chronic illnesses, including rheumatoid arthritis and fibromyalgia, for decades. Over sixty now, her "normal" and healthy appearance belies the constant struggle it is to accomplish daily tasks. Though she has raised two sons and welcomed many others into her home, she doesn't have a lot to put on a traditional résumé.

Currently, Pat provides spiritual direction to several people, including a woman who lives at a psychiatric halfway house. She and her husband recently "adopted" a young woman who lives with them, who decided to sever abusive and toxic ties with her birth family and take on Pat and her husband's last name. She is also involved in peacemaking circles in the Seattle juvenile criminal justice system. I told Pat that if there ever were a "heart and relationship work résumé," hers would be brimming.

In light of Laura's and Pat's stories, we can take heart that living within physical limits can be fertile ground for creativity, emotional transformation, and connection to others. It can expand our imaginations and our hearts, make us ask questions we would never ask otherwise, and show us parts of God that we would never see without our limits. That being said, I would never say that God *caused* an illness or disability *so that* a person might fulfill some bigger purpose. Others disagree; Joni Eareckson Tada, for example, says that God intended for her to become a paraplegic, and made her to be in a wheelchair, so that she could eventually pioneer her ministry to disabled people around the world.[7] Such thinking reads more into God's intentions and workings than I believe is possible given our partial human perspective. We can at the very least, however, trust that God is present and will surprise us with good things, whatever shape—narrow or wide—our life takes.

LIVING WITHIN LIMITS

When my friend Erika was pregnant with her third child, she developed a painful condition where the pelvic bones separate too much. For months, she couldn't climb stairs or lift a laundry basket. Getting in and out of the car the wrong way left her in misery for hours, sometimes days. The strongest memory she has of that season is of sitting in a rocking chair by a big front window in her living room. Erika had never been forced to physically stop like that in her whole life. Some wise mentors counseled her "to be okay with just sitting," she told me—"to feel okay if all I can do, even spiritually, in a day was just sit for ten minutes with Jesus. Not even pray."

Though she could have done without the pain, Erika reflects that parts of that "season of quiet" were a gift. She practiced rest and presence. She tuned in to God in new ways. She was, like the psalmist, made to lie down in green pastures and led beside still waters (Psalm 23). "I very much felt it defined that apparently these are my limits," she said. "This is the small box I was put in. It was nice to know—this is your box."

After Erika gave birth, the pain eventually went away. But she was changed: "I wasn't sure I was returning to the person I was before." She had to learn anew what her body could handle and beyond that—in an intense season of parenting three young children—what she had the mental and emotional capacity for. "I hadn't been good at it, but I've become better at creating quiet spaces for myself," she said. "It's been a process of learning to walk again."

Not all of us will recover from our pain. And many people who are hurting or sick still have responsibilities (in Erika's case, children) that must be met. Some of us don't have the help of family, friends, government programs, or churches and have to work simply to pay bills and provide for our families, even when our bodies should be resting. We need to consider the ways that our society lets some people fall through the cracks, the ways it isn't structured for wholeness. We need to address these systemic problems so all of us can get the rest we need.

But even people who do have the resources to scale back might not dare consider it. The reason goes back to our faulty belief that bodies are secondary to other, more important parts of our selves. If our bodies are simply shells that house our real selves as we go about other, nobler pursuits, then focusing on self-care and prioritizing the needs of our bodies appears misguided and selfish. It would be more worthwhile, more holy even, to deny our bodily limits and press onward, not heeding the pain.

I've come to realize that the relentless voice urging me to push on is not the voice of God. God says, through Jesus, "Come to me, all you that are weary and are carrying heavy burdens, and I will give you rest" (Matthew 11:28). God set bounds on the Israelites' work, building a day of rest into the rhythm of the week, the rhythm of creation (Exodus 20:8-11). And God, through Jesus' incarnation, shows us that the goal of life isn't to transcend our bodies and their limits, but to be fully human within them.

Like Erika had to do while recovering post-partum, people with chronic illnesses must learn to live differently. Our bodies aren't what they used to be. We have better days and worse days, stretches of improvement and setbacks. How can we lean into seasons of forced inactivity and lift them up as our own "sabbaths" (or, maybe more accurately, "sabbaticals," since they often span months, not days)? What does it mean, in our own circumstances, to listen to and honor our bodies and their needs? How can we build rhythms of rest into our lives, affirming that it's okay sometimes just to sit and rock?

We must also realize, though, that limits are not static. Sometimes, as we gradually figure out what habits, treatments, and forms of self-care bring relief, a space opens for more activity. And yet we might be scared to do anything more for fear that the scaffolding around this fragile space will all come tumbling down. Kimberly told me that as she learned to live within her new limits, she got stuck, at one point, in a "cesspool of limitation." She had to tell herself that she was still capable, that she could still push gently in the direction of her heart's desires, whereas previously she might have been driven by obligation or ego, needing to prove things to the outside world. (Indeed, sometimes having less energy or less physical capacity forces us to consider what is really important to us; it crystalizes our calling because we just can't do all the extras.)

Instead of seeing limits as a wall, it might be more helpful to see them as a rubber band. They are flexible, but, pushed too far, we hurt ourselves. When we push, we also need to give ourselves the space to recover, to "bounce back." As part of ministry training some years ago, Erika received the wise advice that though she may have seasons of above-average activity, for every peak, she needed to have an equal amount of low. We need rest to balance our work. We can give ourselves grace in the times of trial and error, as we are learning a new normal. And we can take the risk, sometimes, of trying something new and different.

Not having a five-thousand-channel universe might not be the end of the world. Having just one narrow channel might not be either. According to the poet and farmer Wendell Berry,

8

THE CRAFT OF SUFFERING

*L*abor with my first child started days before his delivery, with a string of nights when I woke up every fifteen to twenty minutes to a tightening that started in my pelvis and rippled up my belly until I was panting with pain. I knew what was happening. We had taken a childbirth class and I had read the books. My uterus was contracting to open up my cervix. My body was getting ready to push a baby out.

Early Saturday morning, December 7, 2013, I finally got fed up with the night labor and made the call to head to the hospital. I was dilated enough to be admitted to the birthing unit, but things didn't go quickly. As I walked the halls with my mom and husband, took a shower, and ate breakfast, I groaned every few minutes, trying not to "brace against the pain" but instead working to "make friends with the heavy feeling of release," as one birthing handout instructed.

I *tried* to do this. But I had one big fear about childbirth, one I had already vocalized to the group of couples taking our childbirth class: "I'm afraid I'm going to poop while the baby is coming out." I said it again to Matt that morning in the hospital as labor slogged along ever so slowly and I grew more exhausted with each wave of pressure and pain: "I'm worried something is going to fall out of me!!" He replied, "Um . . . yeah, that's what's supposed to happen."

Midmorning, our midwife, Gayle, came to check in. She was concerned that, at the rate I was going, I would be facing another night of labor, and then be too exhausted to push at the end. So she suggested Pitocin, a drug that would increase the intensity of contractions to speed up the labor.

At this point, I had my idea of what labor was supposed to be—I wanted to have a natural, unmedicated childbirth with no interventions. Interventions, I had read, often lead to more interventions. Pitocin increases the intensity of labor, which increases the pain, which makes an epidural more likely, which makes a cesarean more likely. I realized then, with the possibility of intervention looming, that I had been trying to maintain control over what was happening in my body. One way or the other, though, I was about to lose control. I could either "make friends with the heavy feeling of release" and allow my bottom to open to let things fall out, or I could hold it in and eventually need interventions, losing control that way.

We asked Gayle to give us another hour before we decided, and then my husband, mom, and I prayed together. As we asked for wisdom and for labor to progress, I began sobbing. The tears, I think, were a physical manifestation of an internal shift. In that moment I finally gave in to the wild, primal process happening in my body. I stopped holding back and instead let the waves come over me without resistance. I tried to go "floppy soggy"[1] and melt into my husband, my mom, the chair, or whatever was supporting me.

After the hour, Gayle came back to check my progress. I was six-to-seven centimeters dilated—farther than she expected.

We decided to hold off on Pitocin and give my body some more time to do what it was doing. Not even a couple hours later, I gave birth to a 10-pound, 7-ounce, 22.5-inch-long baby, with no medical interventions.

I won't mince words. Childbirth hurts. For me, it's also terrifying, no matter how many times I've been through it (three, now). Each time I transition to pushing, my teeth chatter, I sob uncontrollably, and I want nothing more in the world than to stuff the baby back in my belly and avoid the feeling of being rent open from the inside, tissues stretching and tearing, blood and water and baby breaking forth. I'm not one of those women who will talk about having a "lovely" and "beautiful" childbirth. I don't want to do it ever again.

Having experienced it, though, I can see a poetic parallel between childbirth and the rest of life. The suffering that is childbirth required of me a surrender which took several days, with the first baby, to give myself to. I had to let go of my preconceptions of birth—of how it would feel, how long it would take, and the steps in between—and simply be present to each contraction, letting each one fully do its work without worrying about how many had passed or how many there were to go. I had to let go of rational control over my own body and allow an intuitive, animal consciousness to take over. My husband will tell you that my roars during pushing could have bested a lion's, had I met one in that state. To get through labor and make it to the other side intact, I had to shift from resisting the pain—"bracing" myself against it—to "making friends" with it. The pain was not something to back away from, but to melt into. It was not my enemy, but a helpful "heavy feeling of release" that would get my baby out of my womb and into my arms.

"No matter how we are born, we all enter the world through breaking," writes pastor Lee Ann Pomrenke in her article on God as mother.[2] Life begins with a mother's suffering and continues with other forms of suffering peppered throughout. What I learned, in childbirth and in chronic pain, is that it is more fruitful to not resist it but to be present to it. The principle cannot be applied uniformly. When suffering results from injustices caused by human-made institutions, it is right to resist and subvert the structures that cause it. And being present to suffering doesn't mean that we welcome or seek it, or call it "good." Yet when suffering comes and breaks us apart, as it inevitably will—whether because of corporate or individual crookedness, or for no known reason, as part of the inscrutable processes of the universe—we do have choices. As Parker Palmer explains, the breaking can result either in a breaking *apart*, where we shatter into a million tiny pieces, as a brittle vase would, or it can result in a breaking *open* to new life, as a seed cracks for a sprout to emerge.[3]

The Christian community often approaches suffering as a problem to be solved. We stumble over ourselves trying to assign meaning or purpose to tragedy. In the wake of the horrific Sumatran tsunami at the end of 2004, which killed at least a quarter-million people, for instance, many Christians publicly came to God's defense, working hard to reconcile God's omnipotence with God's boundless love. Today, in the era of a deadly coronavirus, we ask the same questions: If God had the power to stop this, and God loves us so much, then why didn't he? How could God allow this? We ask these questions over and over in our own personal tragedies too. Where was God when I needed God the most? Does God care, if he lets me go through *this*?

There is a place for theodicy, but I'm not here to defend God or make the puzzle pieces fit right. Such rationalizing can skate on the surface of the real work we are called to sink into in the face of suffering. Instead of answering the whys, which can be a form of resistance, the more crucial task, I believe, is to let the suffering work on us. We want to emerge not as brittle, shattered beings, but seedlings broken *open*, capable of giving and receiving life, in spite of—or perhaps because of—our suffering.

The metaphor of opening up to pain in childbirth falls apart at some point, because childbirth has an endpoint, and it is visibly fruitful in that a baby results. Most suffering is not so tidy. Is it helpful, or even possible, to be present to suffering when nothing seems to result but more suffering? I think so. I hope so. The apostle Paul speaks of suffering as part of the "groaning of creation" undergoing the pains of childbirth as we eagerly await redemption (Romans 8). Can we trust that our own suffering, whatever it may be, is taken up by God into this epic, universal labor of God's deliverance of all creation? Can we give ourselves over to it, instead of resisting and holding back? And if we do give ourselves over, is there a way to come out on the other end intact, whole, hopeful?

HOW TO SUFFER

We have lost the ability to suffer well. With so many technologies and products that ease discomfort, we nearly get by with the illusion that suffering is entirely avoidable. Our society is so focused on this avoidance that slowly, our definition of the good life has eroded from anything substantial, like treating our neighbors well and taking responsibility for our actions. But, as Christina Bieber Lake aptly asks, "when the good life is assumed to be the life that experiences the least amount of suffering and the maximum amount of happiness, how can we learn to handle the suffering we will inevitably experience?"[4]

We don't handle it well. Like my own initial reaction to chronic pain, many of us get angry and indignant. We feel we have not deserved our lot, we envy others' lives from afar, and we refuse to accept our new reality. Anger and denial are a normal part of grieving, but we get stuck there. Or we numb our pain with entertainment, shopping, drugs, porn, and more. Yet, as theologian Ephraim Radner has observed, we have a deep thirst to know what suffering is about.[5] In a class once, he mentioned a book by a monk called *The Craft of Suffering*. Afterward he received many requests from students asking, "What is this book? Where can I get it?"[6]

This thirst also manifests itself in the rising interest in Eastern spiritual traditions. Buddhist monk Thich Nhat Hanh, who teaches mindfulness practices in the midst of suffering, recently published a book called *No Mud, No Lotus: The Art of Transforming Suffering*.[7] It has received high ratings on Amazon, with hundreds of reviews, such as these two: "I have stage IV lung cancer and this book helped me immensely." "This book was given to me following the sudden death of our 38-year-old son. Excellent writing that helped ease my pain." His talks on the same subject have hundreds of thousands of views on YouTube. These reviewers and watchers, and many others, are looking for guidance—for a "how to" on suffering. This is vastly different than "how to avoid suffering" or "how to explain suffering." They are asking, rather, "How can I live well, even now?"

The Christian tradition has much to offer on this topic. In recent decades, though, a feel-good, therapeutic version of Christianity has seeped into many of our churches,[8] leaving us with the sense that following Jesus should enable us to experience *less* suffering, more health, and more happiness. This is not, however, what Jesus taught. He said clearly, "If any want to become my followers, let them deny themselves and take up their cross daily and follow me. For those who want to save their life will lose it, and those who lose their life for my sake will save it" (Luke 9:23-24). The apostles also spoke of participating in the sufferings of Christ in order to join in his resurrection (Philippians 3:10; 1 Peter 4:13). Throughout the New Testament, the promise is that suffering is not the final answer but the way to new life nonetheless passes through it, through the cross.

Sarah has multiple chronic illnesses including ankylosing spondylitis (a type of spinal arthritis) and lupus. She has also lived through miscarriage, a complicated pregnancy, the death of a child shortly after birth, and having another child born with congenital heart defects. Sarah understands the gospel through the Catholic tradition and points out that Jesus' body is left hanging on Catholic crosses, unlike Protestant crosses that are empty. "We as Catholics do believe his redemption has won grace for us. Heaven is open. We seek and desire that. . . . [But] we're not there yet. Yes, Jesus rose from the dead, but we haven't yet. We're still going through the life where Jesus says, 'Pick up your cross and follow me.'"

Sarah has found deep meaning in the reflections of St. Alphonsus Liguori (interestingly, he is the patron saint of arthritis), who pioneered what became known as the stations of the cross. In her last pregnancy, Sarah's disease activity became unexpectedly high, manifesting as an intensely itchy rash and horrible leg pain caused by vasculitis. She needed daily injections of blood thinners that left painful bruises all over her abdomen. Yet Sarah let her physical sensations become a vehicle to take her to the cross. She used all the tools in her imagination to feel the cross, "the size, the shape, the smell . . . physically on me, and to hug it."

Spinal arthritis was the most recent manifestation of Sarah's various autoimmune conditions. Her suffering has literally taken the shape of a cross in the rigid joints of her vertebrae. This is her cross, Sarah said, and she bears it with love, through love. Our suffering has the power to bring us into the innermost holy of holies with Jesus, where we join it to his and it takes on new meaning.

What is most comforting to me as I read the Gospels is not that Jesus explains the meaning of our suffering or that my pain "makes sense" in God's cosmic economy.[9] It's that Jesus knows my suffering intimately and is here with me in it. When Jesus encounters a funeral procession in Nain for a man who was a widow's only son, he is "moved with compassion" for the widow and raises up her son (Luke 7:11-17 YLT). When his friend Lazarus dies, Jesus sees Mary's weeping, along with the other mourners,' and is "greatly disturbed in spirit and deeply moved" (John 11:33). Before performing another act of resurrection by raising Lazarus from the dead, he enters with them into the pit of loss and mourning. Before conquering death, Jesus weeps.

It is so important to me that Jesus didn't skip over this step. He didn't jump from death to resurrection but dwelt in the darkness and indeterminacy of Holy Saturday, where so many of us spend our days.[10] On Holy Saturday, death has settled, and we don't know yet when new life will come. God's presence is felt as a gnawing absence, a pit in our stomachs and in our souls. We yearn toward Easter, toward Resurrection, but our hearts are not there yet. We need God to be here now. We need to know that God feels what we feel, in this earthly mire of genocides, pandemics, and climate disaster, before we can allow God to lead us—drag us, maybe—out of the pit and onto the rock (Psalm 40:2). In other words, we need to know that God knows the pit, knows how to suffer. And we need to know, as Corrie ten Boom's sister Betsie said, that "there is no pit so deep that He is not deeper still."[11]

This, also, is what comforts me. Jesus stayed in the pit, but he was not obliterated by the darkness that encroaches here. He emerged from the other end, scarred, yes, but whole. He gave himself to the suffering set before him, and it did not break him to pieces but rather opened him to new life. This is my hope—that there is light at the end of this tunnel of death. That when I have lost everything that makes me who I am, I will still remain, because I am held up by something more solid than my self, than my body, than my very consciousness. I am held up by a love as strong as death (Song of Solomon 8:6).

CHOOSING THIS LIFE

Suffering can feel like death, a pain that swallows us whole. As if we touch a hot stove, our initial reaction is to jerk away. My Philosophy 101 professor in college talked about how she got past that reflex when she'd had intense abdominal pain once, which turned out to be appendicitis. Her impulse was to flee, to feel the pain as little as possible. But at some point, she got curious about the fire that was her pain. She let her mind stay in that searing spot, instead of darting away, and asked, "What is the texture of this pain? Where is it, exactly? How does it move through my insides? What are its edges?" She found, as she stayed present, that it was not as all-consuming as she thought. It had a boundary. It was contained to a certain area. She could hold it.

Maybe my professor had above-average mental capacities, being a philosopher and all. But I think we will all find, after we've been around the block enough, that suffering has its edges. It demands its pound of flesh, yes. But after paying our dues, we find—miraculously—that we are still alive.

Hannah Coulter, in Wendell Berry's novel by that name, loses her first husband, Virgil, to World War II. Her grief, she thinks, will knock her over, render her numb. Slowly, though, Hannah begins to feel little happinesses: "the baby, sunlight, breezes, animals and birds, daily work, rest when I was tired, food, strands of fog in the hollows early in the morning, butterflies, flowers. The flowers didn't have to be dahlias and roses either, but just the weeds blooming in the fields, the daisies and the yarrow."[12] Life calls to her.

After some time, life's call comes through the love of another man, Nathan, who eventually becomes Hannah's second husband. At first, she is reluctant to give herself to a life that contains inevitable suffering and loss, uneven and unpredictable in its distribution of joy and sorrow: "To turn to Nathan, to look to him, would be to give my life to the world again. A burnt child shuns the fire."[13] But she does, over time. "I began to trust the world again," she reflects, "not to give me what I wanted, for I was sure that it could not be trusted to do that, but to give unforeseen goods and pleasures that I had not thought to want."[14]

It took many long months for me to crawl through the pit that I fell into while in the worst of my pain. I had to work through anger and denial, depression, and finally, acceptance. I recognize now that these are all parts of the grieving process.[15]

When I came out, I looked around and found I was in a different place. "Normal" was different. I couldn't take long walks. I had to ration any kind of physically strenuous activity. The things people said in church sounded different. What did it mean that Jesus offers us abundant life (John 10:10)? That his yoke is easy and his burden light, when my body was so achy, so dragged down? I squinted to recapture that vision of God I used to have, the God I could trust, to whom I once sang with abandon, "Take myself and I will be, ever, only, all for thee." But I saw mostly shadows and haze.

Yet, I was still alive. Like Hannah Coulter, I began to savor small pleasures. The silken edge of a warm bath rising up my skin. Homemade butternut squash soup in our cozy apartment on a nippy fall evening. Riding the Green Line to graduate school and observing its motley crew of riders. Life was interesting and surprising. Some of it was not what I had expected or wanted, but—slowly—I could say again that it was good.

Around this time, I heard a sermon in church with a six-word takeaway that has stayed with me all these years: "Choose what you did not choose." Life brings us into circumstances we cannot control, that we would never have chosen. I would never choose to have chronic pain as a twenty-two-year-old. I did not choose to grow up in an immigrant family with undocumented parents. My husband and I did not choose to conceive a third baby and be plunged again into the up-to-your-eyeballs, 24/7 work of infant care. But this is my life, the only life I have. I can choose to live it, to be fully present. Or I can reject it, living instead in a past long gone or a future that may never come. "We have to stick with the life that is ours, with its limits, edges, bumps, and filling," writes Ephraim Radner. "By passing through it steadfastly, we learn deeply and we gain wisdom."[16]

ROCKABYE

I would never choose to suffer. Yet what would I be, how would I live, without it? Before having chronic pain, as a teenager and college student, I felt invincible. I thought I was above the principles that govern other peoples' lives, that I was clever enough to evade massive tragedy. I knew, theoretically, that I could die at any time. But I lived as if I would not, at least not for a long while. I was convinced of my own mastery over fate. In my own idealistic, "I'm-going-to-change-the-world" way, I bought into the American dream.

Living with chronic pain has humbled me. I know now that I cannot, by sheer force of will, or faith, or obsessively Googling the heck out of every problem, mold life according to my intentions. I make choices within a set of constraints—my body, my limited span of years, the people whom I am responsible for, who are in turn responsible for me. These givens will, now or later, cause me pain. My body will fail. I will get sick and die. The bodies of those I love will also fail, and I will lose them. This knowledge, once theoretical but now slicing through my marrow, is a source of sorrow. Even as I have and hold, I know I will one day let go and lose. There are physical capacities and people I've already lost. Yet this knowledge also makes life precious. It wakes me up. Knowing it will not last, that it is given and can be taken, I say, "Thank you."

"Is there something about being healthy and well that prevents us from deepening our vision of the world, that keeps us from sensing God's presence in all of life?" asks Stephanie Paulsell. "Perhaps there is. Perhaps suffering makes us more attentive to the miracle of this world. Simone Weil believed that only those who have known both joy and suffering could 'hear the universe as the vibration of the word of God. Joy alone is not enough.'"[17] Even as I affirm these words, I am wary of saying that we *need* suffering to pay attention, to wake up to God. My Christian sensibilities lead me to resist suffering at some basic level; this is not how it should be, right? Could God have really intended that we go through certain terrible ordeals in order to become who we were meant to be?

I've been taught that pain and suffering are not God's plan A; they only entered the world as a result of the Fall. I question this narrative and am compelled by theologies that allow that certain forms of death and pain have been around since the beginning, as part of God's created order. Plant death, bacterial death, animal death—even human death?—are part of the way things are. This perspective helps me accept the suffering that comes to me, particularly bodily suffering through disease or deterioration. Holding to the idea that my body is not how it should be makes me resist the pain. I pray or wish it away. I look to past or future wholeness, rather than learning to be whole in the present.

I don't have answers about what God intended. What I know is that suffering is inescapable in this life and it is futile to try to avoid it. I also question whether it is helpful to try to find the meaning behind the suffering we endure, to try to figure out "God's plan." Are we then trying to explain it away, mounting another form of resistance? I ask a lot of *whys* in my pain, but in the end, the more helpful questions start with *how* and *who*. How will I live now? Who is God for me now? Who am I becoming?

Perhaps we don't need to resist or find meaning behind our suffering, because it takes nothing of ultimate value away from us. "Where, O death, is your victory?" the apostle Paul wrote, "Where, O death, is your sting?" (1 Corinthians 15:55). He proclaimed that death is a momentary passage, leading to the resurrection. What is perishable will be taken up into imperishability, the mortal into the immortal. Our bodies, our souls, our very selves, are held by an everlasting love that is outside of time, outside of death.

One of the things I lost, in suffering, was the ability to say that everything would be okay. Such statements seemed shallow—sugarcoated placebo pills in the face of the horrifying cancer of suffering. What I thought was solid about my faith, about God, was not. "It is not okay!" my soul wailed. "How can *this* be okay?" What I meant by "okay" then was that things would get back to normal. Now I know they might not.

The loss of some of our childlike beliefs, spiritual director Beth Slevcove writes, "is not a journey of moving away from God but part of the journey all of us are on who seek to honestly engage with God throughout a lifetime."[18] Back then, however, I thought I was stepping off the path of faith and into the weeds (down a slippery slope, some would say) of doubt and uncertainty. What I found there, though, was a deeper security, an "okay" born not of knowing, but of unknowing. I don't know what will happen. I may lose the ability to walk again. I may be bedridden, in debilitating pain. One of my children or my husband may get a grave illness. Someone may die. Actually, we all will die. But even then, it will be okay.

If Christianity is to be good news, it must grapple with suffering and say something positive in relation to it, says theologian Karen Kilby. She critiques another theologian, Hans Urs von Balthasar, who seems to give suffering positive value, suggesting that there is something good about suffering in and of itself. Kilby, on the other hand, argues that it's not the suffering itself that has value, but our ability to act in the midst of evil as if it were not. "It makes all the difference," Kilby says, "if that relationship [with suffering] is one of embracing it, as something ultimately bound with love . . . or overcoming it as that which cannot fundamentally touch love."[19]

Jesus shows us that though death cuts deep, almost destroying us, there is a place of being—called forth by love from the very heart of God—that remains. He lived from that place. He rose from the dead out of that place. It is where we came from and where we are going. It is where, if we choose to, we can live from even now. As David wrote, "Even though I walk through the darkest valley, I fear no evil; for you are with me; your rod and your staff—they comfort me. . . . Surely goodness and mercy shall follow me all the days of my life, and I shall dwell in the house of the LORD my whole life long" (Psalm 23:4,6).

Our suffering—whether a result of the natural order or human evil—may seem to annihilate us. Even so, we who follow Jesus believe that because he loves us, and we belong to him, our lives are "hidden with Christ in God" (Colossians 3:3). Knowing this, we don't have to fear or resist suffering. We are freed to walk through it, trusting we will make it to the house of the Lord, into the heart of Love, on the other side.

I've gone through three labors now, learning to feel the pain, to make friends with the heavy feeling of release. I'm here, at the other end, holding a month-old baby, velvety head fresh with the new-human smell, fresh from God. My belly is crisscrossed with dark stretch marks. My bottom has torn and healed over. I'm here scarred, but whole. I sing to my newborn the popular Shawn Mullins song of the 1990s, "Lullaby": "Everything's gonna be all right. Rockabye, rockabye." And I know it's true, not because I'm promised he'll be healthy, or that he'll even live to adulthood. He'll suffer. Probably a lot. Everything's gonna be all right, though, because I love him with that same everlasting love that I'm loved with. He came into being by that love. He'll leave the world in that love. God loved him into life. God's love will cocoon him, even beyond this life.

I choose this life, this life I would not have chosen. I give myself—and my babies—over to God in the unknowns of this life. Everything's gonna be all right.

9

A DIFFERENT WHOLENESS

*C*hronic illness is trauma.[1] My own pain, as it dragged on, was an ongoing, low-level trauma that wore a rut into my body, my brain, my very sense of self. The fact that it had no foreseeable end added to my suffering. Psychiatrist Bessel van der Kolk explains that "situations become intolerable if they feel interminable."[2] The nonstop pain made me want to jump out of my skin and away from my inflamed muscles and joints. But there was no escape. I could not run away from my own body. So instead, I dissociated.

Dissociation is a common response to imminent threats. For early humans, whose main threats were predators like lions, the three options were fight (try to kill the lion), flight (run away as fast as you can), or freeze (play dead or go numb in order to not feel the pain of the attack).[3] Freezing was the last-ditch option if you couldn't fight or run away. And freezing is essentially dissociating—turning off the sensing, feeling parts of your brain so it doesn't hurt as much. Psychologists also call this *depersonalization*.[4]

All of us who have made it to adulthood have dissociated to some degree. Though we come into the world as infants fully present, reaching eagerly for every dirt clod and orange slice, at some point, violence is done to us. Something cuts through that seamless integrity between inner and outer life, between various parts of our selves. We discover, slowly or terribly abruptly, that the world is not a safe place. Even our bodies are not safe.

Threats lurk on all sides. We receive messages from society that what we are is not enough, that we won't be "accepted into the tribe" unless we produce, overcome, and compensate for our vulnerabilities by feigning competence and self-sufficiency. In the United States, people of color, particularly African Americans, also receive the message that their existence, just because of the color of their skin, is unwanted, even a threat. They must work extra hard to prove themselves as worthy in a society skeptical of their worth. All these messages undermine our sense of identity, which is so rooted in the need to belong. We also encounter death and suffering—in our communities where fear and greed drive oppression and violence, in our families where grandparents age and even the young die untimely deaths, in our bodies racked by disease.

At some point, it seems safer not to reach out, not to fully inhabit this fragile flesh and bone. Better, instead, to freeze, to self-protect. In this book we've looked at some of the freezing mechanisms that keep us from being fully present in our bodies, especially when our bodies are suffering. Whether in the legacy of Gnosticism, in our misconceptions of healing, in modern medicine's bent to compartmentalize and control various body parts, or in women's experiences of pain and oppression, we see the same pattern: Stop feeling. Get out of the body or at least try to control it. Cover over the limits, vulnerability, and potential for suffering which the body represents.

All of this "freezing" is understandable—being in a body hurts. Yet continuously walling ourselves off from pain, from the truth of our bodies, comes at great cost. "While numbing (or compensatory sensation seeking) may make life tolerable," van der Kolk writes, "the price you pay is that you lose awareness of what is going on inside your body, and with that, the sense of being fully, sensually alive."[5] As we disconnect from the discomfort, we also lose touch with the very things that will lead to healing.

Psychologist and sex educator Emily Nagoski gives the example of sexual trauma. Survivors often freeze in the moment of assault, whether it is a one-time incident or repeated abuse, and afterward stay locked in that freeze. But, she notes, "survival is not recovery."[6] While dissociating from the body might have been the natural, needed response at the time, recovering requires coming back home to the body, allowing the body to unfreeze and complete the stress cycle.

One of the unfreezing therapies Nagoski highlights is body-based work, such as sensorimotor therapy. She quotes one practitioner who says, "How do we work with the organic intelligence of the body to heal? Instead of managing what comes up from the body, we work with it, trusting its purpose and direction." This could mean allowing your body to tremble, shake, cry, or curl up. "Your body knows what to do," she says.[7] Trust it. This is not easy, when we've been taught, since before we had words, to distrust the body. That vacating it was the best chance for survival, even for sanctity. It is also hard to trust the body when it becomes a source of pain and confusion, as during chronic illness.

Our culture, including church culture, has been in permanent survival-freeze mode, perhaps since the beginning of the human story, when the first cosmic trauma was inflicted through the Fall. But we don't need to be there anymore. We can come home to our bodies. We can recover. We can be whole.

It seems preposterous, I know. Being in a body is just as dangerous and painful as it has always been. How do we come home to something that could—and does—hurt? Why would we now think it's okay? What's changed?

What's changed is that God is here, now. Jesus came to be one of us, in sweat and blood and gasps of pain. He is still one of us now, carrying our aches and cries in his own body. He was nearly obliterated by the heaviness of this life, ground down into the earth and into Sheol, the pit. But he is here, meeting us, past the point where we've given up and we thought it couldn't get any worse. Like a first responder on the scene of a terrible accident, attending to someone very close to death, he says, "Stay with me. Stay present. I am here."

Jesus is the antidote to our dissociation.

People who are frozen in trauma are shut down. "Your heart slows down, your breathing becomes shallow, and, zombielike, you lose touch with yourself and your surroundings," van der Kolk writes.[8] To recover, "we must . . . live fully and securely in the present."[9] In other words, to heal from trauma we must be present and connected—alive in our bodies, in the safe presence of someone who shares our pain and who helps us hold our pain in new ways, ways that don't obliterate us.

Therapists specialize in this work, and for that they play a critical role in society. But before we had words or tools to describe trauma, Jesus was already doing the work of trauma recovery. He remains with us through our pain, our Holy Saturdays in between death and resurrection.[10] He stands with us in the shadow of death, even as the scars on his body witness to the possibility of resurrection. He looks us in the eyes, unafraid of our demons, and says, "You are safe with me. We are together now." When our skittish hearts recoil from all that being a body—being human—entails, Jesus says, "Notice. Breathe. Something new is coming."

Because Jesus lives fully human, fully present in a body, we can too.

ONED TO GOD

In the garden, when Adam and Eve ate the fruit and their eyes were opened, they knew at once the danger of their human existence. At that moment, something was rent apart in their body-soul unity. I wonder if it felt like an out-of-body experience, watching themselves move the fruit to their lips, all the while saying, "Noooo!" In the face of trauma, they dissociated. They froze. They stepped away from their bodies, away from their exposed nakedness, and covered up with fig leaves. This was a tragic separation, the first step in a long, grueling spiral of becoming less-than-human, less-than-whole. But they didn't just separate from their bodies.

As the cool evening breezes blew in, God came walking in the garden to be with Adam and Eve. Hearing the sound, they hid. They ran from the gaze of a loving God for fear of being seen as they now saw themselves—naked, guilty, ashamed. They chose to be apart from God because it was too uncomfortable to be seen up close. Perhaps they worried that God would reject them, so they made the first move. They turned away from God, going their own way rather than staying put. They chose not to wait for God, not to open up about what they had done, not to walk with God in vulnerability and trust.

The rest of the Bible tells the story of what happened after this first trauma—and what God has been doing ever since to heal the rift. "Salvation," writes poet Scott Cairns, "is a continuous process of being redeemed; it is our recovery from our chronic separation from God, both *now* and *ever*, and it includes our becoming increasingly aware of Who our God is."[11]

I love this idea of salvation as recovery from our chronic separation from God. It makes clear that we are gravely ill, but not because we live in vulnerable bodies. It is because we aren't joined as we should be to the God who gives us life. Healing from this illness requires returning to God, or better yet, realizing that God has already come to us in the incarnation of Jesus Christ. Healing is receiving his presence in the here-and-now. Salvation isn't about going up to heaven and escaping our bodies and this world. It's about joining with Jesus in the work he is doing right now, in our stuttering tongues and awkward limbs. Our bodies—at once ghastly and glorious—are Christ's hands and feet.

This is how God saves us: in the incarnation of Christ, he joins himself to us, even in our less-than-whole state. For every step we take away from him, he takes a step nearer. We rejected our bodies as God made them, but God became a human body to be with us in our broken bodies. We denied our vulnerability, but God made himself vulnerable to suffering, pain, and death. We turned away, but God reached out his arms toward us. We divided ourselves from God, God made himself one with us. Atonement, notes Cairns, comes from combining the words at-one-ment, and "was coined in the sixteenth century for the express purpose of reinfusing our theologies with a more vivid awareness of *how* it is that Christ saves us— He joins Himself to us."[12]

If we are to accept this at-one-ing work of Christ, it means we must stay put, stay present when it would be easier to flee to an ethereal reality apart from pain and physical encumbrances. We can only receive Christ as the bodies that we are. Spiritual director Tara Owens was taken aback once when she heard this from the mouth of a monk offering her the Eucharist, "Receive what you are, the body of Christ."[13]

I receive Christ's body too. Here I am, at the Communion rail, holding my two-month-old baby. My husband leads the other two boys up. The five-year-old kneels dutifully while the two-year-old hangs monkeylike from the rail and stares hungrily at the bread coming around. I know he will probably reach out for it and then ask loudly, "What you eating, Mama?" The priest stops in front of me and puts a crumbly, golden piece in my hand. "The body of Christ, given for you." I hurriedly put it into my mouth and chew, because the cup is already here. "The blood of Christ, shed for you." Other times, I have heard, "The blood of Christ, the cup of salvation." If we use Cairns's words, we might also say, "The blood of Christ, the cup of our recovery from our chronic separation from God." Or, to use the language of Nagoski, "The blood of Christ, the cup of our unfreezing. The cup of our reassociation."

Here I am, taking Christ's body into my own. I am chewing Jesus. The enzymes from my saliva and the acids in my stomach are dissolving Jesus into sugar and nutrients that travel through my blood and get used by my cells for energy and growth. Jesus is coursing through my body. He is nourishing my sleep-deprived brain where thoughts feel like cotton candy—wispy bits of nothing that melt away upon contact. He is here in the interstices of my too-tight neck and back, which sometimes spasm with pain. He is here in my pelvis, still recovering from childbirth, still sore when I cough and sneeze. This is my body, a body that Jesus joins himself to. I receive Christ, and so I receive my own body. I am becoming whole, becoming *one* with Christ. As I masticate my risen Lord, I also digest the truth that the fourteenth-century anchoress Julian of Norwich spoke so tenderly, "Our life is all grounded and rooted in love, and without love we may not live . . . we are endlessly oned to Him in love."[14]

BODIES AND BREATHING

In my early adult years, I thought I was whole because I was healthy, mobile, and able to do what I wanted. Now I realize that this kind of wholeness is fleeting. It is a superficial wholeness based on our ability to perform and conform to our society's idea of normal. Theologian Deborah Beth Creamer writes that disability is an open minority that any of us might join at any time, especially as we get older. "It has been suggested that it makes little sense to try to distinguish between able and disabled," she said, "but rather that any difference is simply between disabled and temporarily able-bodied."[15]

Since physical health and ability are temporary, they cannot be the markers of true wholeness, because they aren't really *who we are*. Parker Palmer describes the jack pine, its jagged outline standing against the elements of wind, drought, cold, heat, and disease, and how it speaks of wholeness, "an integrity that comes from being who you are."[16] In a similar way, who we are has to be what remains after we have been ravaged by the winds, droughts, cold, heat, and diseases of life. We are still standing (or sitting, or lying). We are still here as embodied souls, ensouled bodies. Our limbs might be knotted and gnarly, our shoulders stooped, our skin scarred and wrinkled. But learning to live in these wind-torn bodies, the only ones we will ever have, is its own kind of beauty, its own kind of healing.

We cannot separate out our bodies and our selves, try as we might.

Like my husband, I have had spells of insomnia. On the nights when my breath comes shallow and my brain keeps whirring along, keeping my body from sinking into the depths of sleep, I wish I could push a button and simply disconnect. It would be so nice if the stresses of the day and my anxiety for tomorrow didn't weave knots into my shoulders and twitches into my legs. If my body could reset without my heart and mind having to as well.

But, as Stephanie Paulsell reminds us, we don't just *have* bodies. We *are* bodies.[17] The pressures on my mind—whether it's my concern that my son's cough will develop into an asthma attack or the worry that I won't meet a deadline—don't happen apart from my body. They are somehow lodged in my cells and tissues, and they keep me awake. To release my body into sleep, I also have to release my thoughts and emotions. I have to reconnect body and mind, tending to both as a whole.

To help him sleep, Matt has been meditating through an app called Headspace. Meditation is similar to yoga, which I'm more familiar with. You focus on your breath, being intentional about each inhale and exhale. You scan your whole body, from toes to scalp, noticing what is going on in every part, whether tension or pain. You tune in to the physical sensations—the sound of a clock ticking or the feel of the air over your skin. These practices "bring our mind home to our body," writes Thich Nhat Hanh. Breathing with intention brings us down to earth, back to ourselves. "The process of healing begins," Hanh says, "when we mindfully breathe in."[18]

Breathing also has significance in the Christian tradition. In Genesis, God forms man from the dust and breathes life into his nostrils so that he becomes a living being (2:7). The Hebrew word for the spirit of God is *ruach*, which also means "breath" or "wind." In addition, the ancient Jesus Prayer works with the rhythm of breathing: "Lord Jesus Christ" (inhale), "have mercy on me" (exhale). Our breath serves as a reminder of who we are and from whom we come. It grounds us in our identity as God's beloved creatures, dependent on him for mercy.

Our breath may be the one thing that remains constant throughout life. Whether young or old, running marathons or bedridden, we still breathe. When we are stripped of everything else, we still have our breath, a reminder that we are alive and that God is sustaining us. Each breath we take, if we pay attention, can reenact this original impartation of life. *Breathe in:* receive God's gift of life. *Breathe out:* let go of your death clutch on life; know that your next breath comes only from God. *Breathe in:* know that you are God's creature. *Breathe out:* lean on your Creator.

Trauma therapists use breath as a powerful tool. Van der Kolk recalls meeting Annie for the first time. She shuffled into his office, "barely breathing, looking like a frozen bird." He realized he could do nothing until he could help her quiet down:

> Moving to within six feet of her and making sure she had unobstructed access to the door, I encouraged her to take slightly deeper breaths. I breathed with her and asked her to follow my example, gently raising my arms from my sides as she inhaled and lowering them as I exhaled . . . she stealthily followed my movements, her eyes still fixed on the floor. . . . From time to time I quietly asked her to

notice how her feet felt against the floor and how her chest expanded and contracted with each breath. Her breath gradually became slower and deeper, her face softened, her spine straightened a bit, and her eyes lifted to about the level of my Adam's apple.

After about a half hour, van der Kolk felt he had made enough demands on Annie for the day and asked if she would like to come back a week later. She nodded and replied, "You sure are weird."[19]

When we are in pain, paralyzed with fear, or just feeling uncomfortable and distant from our bodies, paying attention to our breath can be a small yet crucial way forward. It can bring us out of anxious headspaces and into the here and now. Maybe our breath will come out as groans. Even then, God's Spirit joins us in releasing those "sighs too deep for words" (Romans 8:26).

As we inhale and exhale, we remember we are God's creatures, enlivened by God's own breath. We are bodies that need to eat and sleep, rest and play. We are God's own; we are Christ's body, "endlessly oned to him in love." In God "we live and move and have our being" (Acts 17:28). When we perform the simple act of breathing, of coming home to our bodies even if it's the only thing we can do, we are becoming whole.

MOSAIC-MAKING

I was at Lincoln Marsh one fall, hashing the whole chronic pain thing out with God for the hundredth time. In the waning light, as the air got nippy, I looked over the cattails and reeds. The vision I had for my life was in pieces. I approached God with the pieces in my hands, wanting him to put them back into their original shape. Every piece was a pet project or dream I didn't know if I'd be able to do with my ongoing pain, or an important aspect of my identity that I couldn't part with: being able to dance, keeping my house clean on my own, going on a walking pilgrimage through Spain. Nothing—who I thought I was, who I thought God was—fit with my reality.

My part of the dialogue involved me desperately sorting through the pieces and trying to line them up so there were no gaping holes or cracks and so that they formed the same picture as before. In my frantic sorting, though, I started to sense God doing something else. He was not interested in lining all the pieces up in a coherent whole—at least not a whole that I could understand. God was holding out his hands underneath mine, even as I clung to the shards. *Let go,* he said. *I will hold them for you. It's okay that your life is in pieces. Be okay with the pieces.*

I heard this, and my heart tightened. Still, I wanted to let go and trust, so I tried to act out in my body what I couldn't do quite yet in my soul. Sitting on a bench overlooking the marsh, I extended both fists with my palms downward and then un-clenched my fingers one by one, opening them wide to the ground. I pictured God's hands catching my pieces. I cried. I breathed. And I went home.

Trauma researchers note that survivors are often stuck in the moment of the traumatic event, unable to reconcile past and present. The fragments of their experience—the smells, the horror and paralysis, the lighting—are replayed again and again in a never-changing present. What trauma patients need is the ability to integrate the traumatic memories into their current life in a way that gives them a sense of completion. Then the experience "stops having a life of its own."[20]

As I clutched the fragments of my life, I was trying to find that sense of integration. But I wanted it to be a wholeness that

I knew, a wholeness not formed out of brokenness. That fall afternoon at Lincoln Marsh, I felt God nudging me toward a different wholeness. A true wholeness that accounts for the pain and accepts the pieces without trying to force them back into a prebroken state. Wholeness must embrace our current brokenness, or it is not wholeness, but nostalgia.

We've internalized from so many sources that to be whole means to go back to some previous state of purity. But it's impossible to go back. Those who have survived sexual trauma know this. They live with the flashbacks and nagging question of, "What did I do to invite this?"[21] Those of us who grew up in evangelical purity culture get the message that once we screw up—or once life screws us up—we can't be "pure" and "whole" any longer. Being sexually intimate before marriage is like being a piece of duct tape that gets stuck to a surface and then peeled off, my high school youth pastor said. The more times you do it, the less sticky you become. Once you're broken, like Humpty Dumpty, you just can't be put back together again. The idea bleeds into other areas of our embodied lives, including our experiences of illness. We think our bodies are forever faulty, dysfunctional, no longer "blessed."

But we are not pieces of duct tape. Or Humpty Dumpty. We are living beings with God's breath in us. Morsels from the Creator and Redeemer of human life, who gave his body to one himself to us, are coursing through our veins. He can transform our brokenness.

In his work with trauma survivors, van der Kolk discovered a technique called EMDR (eye movement desensitization and reprocessing), which involves having a patient revisit a traumatic memory while tracking the therapist's moving finger. He surmises that the rapid eye movements bring the mind to a state similar to REM sleep, where it is able to make distant associations and connect fragments of traumatic memories with other, more recent memories. In one very successful case, he noted, "the process freed something in her mind/brain to activate new images, feelings, and thoughts; it was as if her life force emerged to create new possibilities for her future."[22]

When I embodied the act of letting go, releasing the fragments of my life into God's hands, I was—symbolically, at least—stepping out of the never-ending present of my pain and allowing new possibilities to emerge. I was trusting God to hold the pieces of who I was, to make use of the brokenness. Now, looking back, I can see how the pieces are coming back together in a new way, forming a different, but equally meaningful, picture. But that afternoon at Lincoln Marsh, I first needed to free my imagination away from the fixation on "going back to normal" (and maybe I needed a few good nights of busy REM sleep; I was not sleeping well then). Van der Kolk writes, "Seeing novel connections is the cardinal feature of creativity; as we've seen, it's also essential to healing."[23]

We recently made our first mosaic as a family. We used glass clippers and broke several amber, green, and black wine bottles into little pieces. We scraped the edges of each piece on a sanding block to smooth the too-sharp edges and stuck them to a piece of plywood around a mirror in a wave-like design. Our mosaic mirror hangs over an old wine barrel that my husband turned into a sink. It is more beautiful, I think, than the wine bottles themselves. It speaks to our human creativity in turning broken shards into a different whole. This, in turn, points to our creative God, who partners with us in doing the same thing with our lives. If we can first let go of the pieces.

PART OF A WHOLE

Whole Foods has this hashtag #MakeMeWhole, which I see beneath pictures of artisanal cheese and artfully piled blueberries on banners throughout the store. I always feel slightly sheepish and defiant shopping here, knowing I am fulfilling the stereotype of the health-conscious, middle-class mom. This mom buys organic to keep her kids pure and assuages her guilt about her role in the overconsumption of the world by consuming more expensive, "socially responsible" stuff at stores like this. As I push my cart around and ogle at all the gorgeous, overpriced displays, I want to wear a shirt that says, "I'm not *that mom.*" And yet, I am.

Even as I appreciate the selection of items that are more responsibly sourced and less chemical-laden, I want to resist Whole Foods' underlying message—that wholeness is a matter of individual consumption. That I can buy my way to wholeness for myself and my family. #MakeMeWhole is focused on "me"— how *I* can take care of *my* family by purchasing natural products. As a side benefit, the store donates a portion of purchases to their philanthropic efforts around the world. But the focus is on my choices as the individual consumer. As if buying organic, fair-trade bananas were enough to be whole.

The word *individual* means "that which cannot be divided." In our North American capitalist society, we like to think that the basic unit of society is the individual. Individual people making their individual choices that affect their individual lives. But this individualistic mentality is only a recent phenomenon in the long history of humankind, where, more often than not, individuals could only survive as part of a group. In prehistoric times, for instance, a nearsighted person could not survive outside of the tribe. They would be devoured by a lion before seeing it from afar. The hunters with good eyesight, in turn, required the help of others to process and distribute the kill. When one hunter didn't get a catch for a while, he didn't starve because he was part of a group who shared resources—meat, nuts, roots, and berries hunted and gathered by others.

It's easy to see the need for dependence in the example of a small hunter-gatherer tribe, but even today we need countless, often-invisible others to survive. The COVID-19 pandemic reveals this truth. "Flattening the curve" of contagion requires that almost all members of society wash their hands, keep their distance from each other, and comply with the latest public health guidelines. I may not think that my staying home for weeks on end is accomplishing much, but it is part of what keeps an eighty-year-old woman across town from getting sick and dying.

When we look at our individual issues—nearsightedness, cancer, immune insufficiency or hyperactivity, etc., etc.—we can approach healing in two ways. The first way is what we commonly think of: trying to fix our individual bodies so that we can become more independent—see clearly, not get sick, have energy and mobility. It is legitimate to seek healing in this way. But it doesn't always happen, and we shouldn't stop here.

Another way to think about healing is to consider how we rely on each other to compensate for the physical "flaws" any one individual may have. When I couldn't walk much, for instance, my husband carried the laundry up and down the stairs, washed the dishes, and picked up around the house. We joked that he was an extension of me, another set of arms and legs and a back for me to use when my own were not functional. (It gave the "one flesh" language of marriage completely new meaning!) When I was in pain, the illusion that I am an individual independent of others faded and the truth that I need others in order to survive came into focus. In the coronavirus pandemic, we are learning as a global society that preventing the virus's spread requires coordinated action by national and local governments and cooperation from the public, not just individual people trying to protect themselves.

For those who've experienced trauma, connection with a broader community can be an essential part of their healing. "The essence of trauma," writes van der Kolk, "is feeling god-forsaken, cut off from the human race."[24] He goes on to document how collective ceremonies and rhythms, like chanting, dance, and theater, play a crucial role in helping traumatized people reinhabit their bodies. They find new strength and courage in being part of something bigger than themselves. I wonder if this is why protests can be so empowering for those who have been historically oppressed. In a mass of other bodies united to call out injustice, we find we are not alone. Injustice and violence cut us off from humanity, but collective action reunites.

Anthropologist Cara Wall-Scheffler, observing the evolutionary history of humankind, notes that we were only able to survive and thrive because we lived in interdependent groups. She calls this a "selective advantage for community." So-called flaws, she suggests, are opportunities for relationship and grace.[25] In the popular understanding of evolutionary theory, we've internalized a message of "survival of the fittest"—the strongest, healthiest individuals survive. But Wall-Scheffler suggests that it's not healthy *individuals* who survive, but healthy *communities*. If the unit of selection is the community, because lone people (even lone families) cannot make it on their own, then perhaps the word *individual* is not appropriate for a single person. "That which cannot be divided" is the community—we cannot live apart from others. We often try, though, to our own harm.

The individualist mentality has seeped into how we think about faith and salvation as well. Individual people "make a decision" for Christ. But some stories in the Bible blur the line between individuals. When Paul and Silas's jailer asked what he must do to be saved, they replied, "Believe in the Lord Jesus, and you will be saved—you and your household." Then, when the jailer brought them back to his house and set a meal before them, "he was filled with joy because he had come to believe in God—he and his whole household" (Acts 16:31-34 NIV). Here, the basic unit of society—and of saving faith—is the household, not the individual. A household at that time might include slaves, servants, aunts, uncles, cousins, and grandparents— more like a clan or tribe than what we think of in North American society as the "family."

The church where my family worships now is part of the Anglican tradition, which carries on some of this household-based understanding of salvation in their practice of infant baptisms. The child being baptized cannot speak, and so the family speaks on their behalf. They commit to bringing the child up in the way of truth and knowledge of Christ. The congregation, too, agrees to support the family.

My friend Erika has a six-year-old who was recently baptized in the Anglican church (this was Erika and her husband's compromise between believer's baptism and infant baptism). In letting their son undergo baptism, she explained, she and her husband were saying, "We recognize the seed that God has planted in you. We are committed to nurturing that seed and trusting God to make it grow." This is a recognition of our intimate dependence on others—for faith, for life, for salvation. It's not simply a matter of personal decision and willpower. We need others in order to know who God is, and who we are.

For Christians, the church provides a tangible community in which we can locate ourselves. But our ultimate healing lies beyond connecting with people in church. We are also cut off from God's creation. We need to find a rhythm not just with our fellow humans, but with all of God's green earth.

HEALING AND THE EARTH

"Oh no, they flooded. Look, the waters stopped at their front steps. Wow, the bridge collapsed." My mom and I were watching an aerial drone video of her neighborhood in southeast Texas in the days following Tropical Storm Imelda, which hit just two years after Hurricane Harvey in 2017. For many, Imelda was Harvey 2.0,[26] a wash of relentless rains that brought catastrophic flooding. My mom happened to be up north visiting me and Matt and our boys this time, leaving my younger brother in the house to weather the storm on his own. (He was a nervous wreck, watching the waters rise and close in on the house.)

Their house didn't get inundated this time, thankfully, but many others did. In my high school hometown, so many were once again ripping up soggy carpet and drywall, sorting through what could be salvaged. The long ordeal of bureaucratic red tape for insurance reimbursements and FEMA support began yet again. As I scrolled through the Facebook updates from my friends in the area, I heaved a deep sigh of frustration and lament. Again!? How could a thousand-year rain event happen every other year? Something was amiss.

In recent decades it has become obvious that the earth we rely on is in a state of chronic illness. Forests that supply much-needed oxygen are catching fire and burning uncontrollably. Land that gives us food is becoming nutrient poor, resulting in deficiencies and illness in those who sustain themselves with the crops harvested from it.[27] Hurricanes, droughts, and heat waves are becoming more extreme and regular events.

The earth, like our bodies, is sending distress signals. Something isn't right about the way we are inhabiting this planet. And just as we cannot barricade ourselves from the vulnerability and suffering of our human neighbors, so we cannot partition ourselves off from the suffering of the rest of creation.

"We know that the whole creation has been groaning in labor pains until now," says Paul, "and not only the creation, but we ourselves, who have the first fruits of the Spirit, groan inwardly while we wait for adoption, the redemption of our bodies" (Romans 8:22-23). Creation groans. We groan. We are part of this big roiling mess. We are part of creation. Our first disobedience and separation at the Fall had consequences not just for human bodies and relationships; the trauma has been reverberating throughout all of God's world. When we do not recognize who we are—siblings with the rest of the created order, the whispering trees, tunneling earthworms, and crashing waves—we all suffer.

There is an "intrinsic connection between positive or negative human action and the flourishing or diminishing of the non-human world," writes theologian Richard Middleton. In Genesis, Cain's violence against his brother Abel spills over to the human-earth relationship, such that the earth "will no longer yield" its crops to Cain (4:12). Later, in the time of Noah, the whole earth floods as a result of the violence and corruption of the humans who live upon it (Genesis 6). Middleton goes on to explore how the prophets, too, elaborate on the idea of "close linkage between the moral and cosmic orders."[28] Isaiah states:

> The earth dries up and withers,
>> the world languishes and withers;
>> the heavens languish together with the earth.
> The earth lies polluted
>> under its inhabitants;
> for they have transgressed laws,
>> violated the statutes,
>> broken the everlasting covenant. (24:4-5)

If our separation from God involved not just other humans but the whole of the cosmos, so too will our redemption bring along the rest of creation.

> The wilderness and the dry land shall be glad,
>> the desert shall rejoice and blossom;
> like the crocus it shall blossom abundantly,
>> and rejoice with joy and singing.
> The glory of Lebanon shall be given to it,
>> the majesty of Carmel and Sharon.
> They shall see the glory of the LORD,
>> the majesty of our God. (Isaiah 35:1-2)

Our healing—our recovery from our chronic separation from God—is not just for us. It's for the trees, the earthworms, and the waves too. The heavens declare God's glory; the sky "pours forth speech" and "declares knowledge" (Psalm 19:1-2). The rocks, too, cry out (Luke 19:40).

How can we pay attention to what creation is saying? How can we tune in to the pain of a groaning creation and recognize the groans as our own? How can we inhabit creation just as we inhabit our bodies—gently, tenderly, noticing, and honoring?

Being out in the natural world is a balm for many. Under a cathedral of trees or in the holy silence of the desert we sense our oneness with all that God has made. We are not alone. We are accompanied in our joy and pain not just by other humans but by daffodils, ladybugs, and sugar maples.

So we tend to the earth as part of our healing. I call my representatives in Congress and beseech them to act on climate change. I plant arugula seeds and mark the days of our COVID-19 shelter-in-place by their growth. I take my children to the forest preserve and point out the mallards quacking in the reeds. I notice new life under these cold prairie skies. I collect in my heart the hints of spring, and—amid a pandemic that separates me physically from other humans—I sense a deeper connection.

10

A COMMUNITY OF
WOUNDED HEALERS

From the time William was a child, he had pain going to the bathroom. He didn't know it was a problem until his parents started taking him to the doctor to do some tests. In his teen and early adult years he lived with the pain until it started to get progressively worse in his thirties. After some internet sleuthing, William realized he had all the symptoms of interstitial cystitis, which for him involves bouts of intense pain caused by small amounts of urine around the bladder.

"My life," William said, "revolves around the bathroom." In every new place, he makes a mental note of the closest bathroom. He has stopped doing activities where he might not be able to get to one for extended periods—flying and taking long car rides, going to the theater, attending sports games. "Many times I can only survive on opioid medications," William said, and even those don't help much, as his body seems unable to metabolize medications, and many leave him with side effects worse than the symptoms they're aiming to alleviate.

William works a relatively high-stress job at a state university but foresees having to leave it and go on disability in the near future. "Barring something miraculous happening, I'm in the twilight of my working years. I'm forty-five. Typically, people who have this condition don't work past their forties. So I am following that pattern." He is worried about being able to support himself after going on disability, as even now—with decent health insurance—he pays a significant amount each year for out-of-pocket medical expenses.

Though he's had some significant relationships, William remains single. At least one of the relationships ended once the other person realized the depths of his health issues. "A lot of what I'm dealing with is so much more complicated when I'm single," he said. "You still have to do the laundry, take care of yourself, and all the daily stuff."

William doesn't tell many people about his illness. "It's difficult to explain and embarrassing. I have something weird, dealing with part of the body that people don't normally talk about," he explained. Being a man also makes it harder. He has a condition that is more common in women, and men are socialized to be less expressive about their pain than woman. "Even my closest friends don't know what it's truly like from day to day," he said. Nonetheless, having a handful of people with whom William can be open about his illness has been crucial to his mental and emotional well-being. "I've discovered there are other people who, even though they are not going through serious issues themselves, have a level of empathy and caring," he shared. "It becomes less of a burden, at least emotionally, when you can talk about your issues with other people."

Though William's close confidants are Christians, the church as a whole hasn't been a place where he can be honest. He has experienced significant anxiety and depression and a deep

crisis of faith because of living with this progressively dete-
riorating and painful disease. "It's not like I've been given a
death sentence," he explained. "But sometimes you wish you
would . . . because that would be preferable to having to live
with it." These are thoughts he can't share in church. "Church
is your country club," he said. "It's not the place to talk about
your problems. People are not accepting when you say you
struggle with your faith because of condition X, Y, Z. I've been
in many different churches. Finding those pockets of supportive people is hard."

MORE THAN A COUNTRY CLUB

Many with chronic illness, like William, find church to be difficult
or unsupportive—not a place where they can bring their suffering. Many speak of healing and supportive relationships with
other Christians, but these are "pockets," as William put it. They
don't reflect the culture of the evangelical church as a whole.

I can relate. Getting ready for church, I try to put on my
smiling, "blessed" face—the one that shows the world I am
truly a beloved child of God. I wipe off the scowl I was giving
my two-year-old for getting maple syrup in my hair. I pretend
I got eight hours of uninterrupted sleep. I assume that people
will think less of me if I come to church disheveled or crabby
or sad. I know this assumption is wrong and stems from my
own insecurities and projections upon others. And yet, if I am
making these projections, I'm probably not alone. It means the
majority of us come to church pretending to be happier than
we really are, creating a culture where it appears that everyone
is just fine—not dealing with pit-in-your-stomach, hole-in-
your-heart issues. And this makes it hard to be the lone person
to raise their hand and say, "Um, yeah . . . I'm really not okay."

Writer Barbara Brown Taylor calls this the "full-sun effect." In the patterns of her own inner life, her soul operated on a lunar calendar, coming up at different times each night and never looking the same two nights in a row. In church, however, she felt compelled to be all sunshine. As a priest, she was troubled to note that people always disappeared from church when their lives were breaking down, whether from divorce, illness, depression, job loss, or alcoholism. She writes,

> I was sorry that the church did not strike these wounded souls as a place they could bring the dark fruits of their equally dark nights . . . even people in no apparent crisis seemed to suffer from the full-sun effect. As enjoyable as it could be to spend a couple of hours on Sunday morning with people who were at their best, it was also possible to see the strain in the smiles, the effort it took to present the most positive, most faithful version of the self. Sometimes I could almost read the truth written out above people's heads: "Please don't believe me. This is only a shard of who I really am." The cost of the pretense was the loss of the real human texture underneath, but since we all thought that was what was expected of us, that was what we delivered.[1]

The full-sun effect, Taylor points out, is a loss—we lose the chance to know each other in the fullness of who we are. We lose the profound wisdom that comes from being present to the brokenness and allowing our eyesight to adjust to see the treasures hidden in the dark. And this kind of wisdom is crucial to our becoming faithful communities of Jesus-followers— communities where the sick, outcast, doubting, and wandering can find a home. Jesus ministered specifically to these people.

You might say that among his disciples, people who were sick, "abnormal," and socially ostracized took center stage. Why don't our churches—particularly our leadership—reflect what Jesus' earliest followers looked like?

It will take a major revamping to make church more than a country club. Perhaps it has to start with creating those "pockets" of safe spaces where people relate to each other in all honesty, whether one-to-one or in small groups. But eventually, we come up against those deep frameworks around which we've built our communal life: our assumptions about normalcy and about the faithful, fruitful Christian life; our conceptions of ministry and giftedness and of who is qualified to be up front. Demolition is needed. We will have to take down some deeply rooted structures.

LISTEN. PERIOD.

Just today I read a friend's email telling me about some hard marital, physical, and emotional things she's going through. As I shut my laptop and went about my morning, the first thoughts that came to mind were: (1) Have they seen a counselor? (2) Has she seen a physical therapist? (3) She should try X treatment. Then I stopped myself. She probably wasn't telling me about her problems so I could solve them. Yet my go-to response was to try to "fix" her.

People with chronic illnesses get a lot of well-intentioned, misguided advice. See this doctor. Drink more water. Eat more vegetables. Avoid gluten. Drink bone broth. Do yoga. Forgive your dad. Relax. Don't try so hard. Try harder. While we know that others are trying to help, the underlying message we receive is that something is the matter with us. We're doing something wrong. What we're experiencing isn't quite right, and we need to get better so that others don't feel so uncomfortable, confused, or threatened around us. When we don't tie up our stories with, "But God is good; he has a plan," or "But I know he'll heal me in his timing," or some other positive note, listeners start to squirm. It's as if they need that positive cap on the experience in order for it to be contained; otherwise they fear that the darkness and suffering will seep over onto them, that they'll catch the pain.

Often, as listeners, if we don't get that happy cap, we try to add our own. We work to find solutions, to make it feel like we've done something. Or we look for a silver lining. Kate Bowler writes that once a well-meaning neighbor came to their door while she was undergoing cancer treatment. The woman reassured Kate's husband that everything happens for a reason.

"I'd love to hear it," he replied.

"Pardon?" she said, startled.

"The reason my wife is dying," he said in that sweet and sour way he has, effectively ending the conversation as the neighbor stammered something and handed him a casserole.[2]

Debi lost her father to an early death. "If one more person said to my mother, 'God can be your husband' or 'Suffering makes us stronger' she would have lobbed them in the head," she said. "We're so quick to say 'God loves you. God will be able to take care of you. God has a plan.' All those things are true, but let them suffer. Let them feel pain. Don't be so quick to say, 'God will fix it.' Because what if he doesn't?"

Learning to listen without fixing and judging is not easy. By judging, I don't only mean judging the person for having negative, difficult, perhaps heretical thoughts or emotions. I also mean judging the situation. We so quickly want to label a situation as "good" or "bad," as part of God's plan or outside of it. But in order to allow people to heal we must practice deep, nonjudgmental listening without an agenda.

I could write an entire book on this topic, but thankfully there already is one. Parker Palmer's *A Hidden Wholeness: Welcoming the Soul and Weaving Community in a Wounded World* outlines how to create "circles of trust" based on the tried-and-true Quaker practice of clearness committees. In this practice a group gathers to help a specific person gain insight into a problem or question or make an important life decision. Committee members ask open and honest questions, questions that make space for the soul to come out of hiding. "An *honest* question," Palmer writes, "is one I can ask without possibly being able to say to myself, 'I know the right answer to this question, and I sure hope you give it to me.'" "What is the biblical solution to this?" is not an honest question, if you already have an answer in mind that you're trying to draw out. Something like, "What past experiences might be useful to you in your current dilemma?" is. "How do you feel about the situation you just described?" is also *open*, whereas, "Do you feel any anger?" is not.[3]

One summer when I was in college, my mom and stepdad seemed on the verge of splitting up. I met up with my friend Katie, one of a few people I consider part of my lifelong clearness committee. We walked countless circles around her Houston subdivision as she listened without judgment and asked clear-eyed questions like, "What do you feel responsible for, and why? How is God leading you?" She reflected back what I said so I had clarity on my own thoughts and reactions. She didn't give me advice. She didn't tell me this was part of God's plan. Yet, because she provided a safe, hospitable space, I was able to dig deep into my own inner resources and sink down to that place where God dwells. I discovered that I had the capacity to be present to the deep brokenness in my family without walling myself off from the pain. I could feel the pain without letting the heaviness push me into the ground.

Katie's listening led toward healing, allowing me to find my way through the forest of family conflict. She could have told me the same things I discovered for myself, but I don't think they would have stuck. Her listening facilitated the soul work that precedes deep, interior transformation. The truths I gained were fully mine. I was able to live them as the unique human being that I am, rather than trying to squeeze myself into another person's understanding of truth. In that Houston subdivision, I walked, with Katie, a few steps closer to wholeness. What soul work do we each need to do in order to provide this kind of listening to others?

PRACTICAL SERVICE

There are other practical ways churches and individuals can walk alongside people with chronic illnesses. I've included a few below, but keep in mind that we are not problems to be fixed, but rather wounded healers whose gifts—and simple presence— are also desperately needed by the church and world.[4]

Meals. I've been a grateful recipient of meal ministries at various churches for the happy reason of having babies. Meal ministries also help those who are suffering—perhaps going through an operation, cancer treatment, or a death in the family. Chronic illness is an indeterminate kind of need, though. How many weeks can you ask for meals before you've used up your "quota"? People with chronic illnesses tend to stop asking for help or being upfront about their true needs for fear of overburdening and burning others out.

If you know someone with a chronic illness, consider cooking up a double batch every once in a while and sharing a meal with them. Or consider keeping a regular rotation of long-term meal recipients at your church. People with chronic illnesses and disabilities—or single moms, for that matter—would benefit.

Medical advocates. When we are chronically ill, we can get stuck in the maze of the medical system. We don't know who to see or what to ask. Sometimes doctors dismiss us because we are too emotional. Debi said, "It's important to have somebody else at your appointment with you. Because you need that support. Somebody to help you fill in the blanks of your story because you forget."

One of my friends called these people "medical advocates." They can help sick people navigate the medical system by driving them to and from appointments, filling out paperwork, being at appointments to be a second voice for the patient, and taking notes. People who are farther along in the chronic illness journey might also serve as advocates, providing a helpful point of reference for those who are just beginning to untangle symptoms and see different doctors.

Presence and physical touch. There is something healing about simply having another warm human body next to yours when you are hurting. We need physical touch to grow and thrive. Babies deprived of touch are at higher risk of behavioral, social, and emotional problems as they grow up.[5] At any age, a simple hug can defuse stress and reset our moods. One of my husband's go-to strategies for breaking up fights among our boys is to tell them to stop and hug each other.

Offering people with chronic illnesses—or anyone who is suffering—the gift of our physical presence (as well as a hug if they want) is a basic way to show care and love. Simply ask if you can hang out and then show up. "The emptiness of the past and the future can never be filled with words," writes Nouwen, "but only by the presence of a human being."[6]

Financial help. This one—like meals—is tricky. How much do you ask for before you use up more than your "share"? Many of us have problems asking for money—even if we desperately need it. This underscores our illusions of independence as Americans and our reluctance to become "recipients," as if this somehow makes us second-class citizens.

Yet, many with chronic illnesses struggle financially, particularly if they are not married and don't have relatives to support them. Their conditions may keep them from holding full-time jobs or perhaps any job. Going on disability might not cover all their needs. They may have trouble even getting disability aid. They end up having to make difficult choices between getting medical care or groceries, paying for medicine or paying the bills. There are no rules to this or any issue related to chronic illness. We can simply follow Jesus' commands as faithfully as we can: "Give to anyone who asks you" (Luke 6:30 NIV) and—I would add—don't be afraid to ask.

Inclusive community events. Laura, the artist who made art out of her hearing loss, told me her condition completely changed how she does church. For a while, she would sit through two worship songs and have to throw up. Then she did some research and realized that one of the symptoms of cholesteatoma is nausea from loud noises. She had to skip the singing and come for the Scripture reading and sermon. It felt at first like a withdrawal from community and pushed Laura to relate to God differently. She realized she could also worship God in listening and silence. So she stopped singing in the choir and got involved in lower-key women's ministry. "Even if you're limited in one way that doesn't mean you're limited in all your senses," she said.

How can we make our gatherings more accessible to those with chronic illnesses, whose abilities to stand or dance or sing or hear may be changed by their condition? How can we make our worship more accessible emotionally to those who have felt isolated by the full-sun effect and crave a space to bring their true emotions, their lament, before God?

We often default to certain activities because they are what we've always done—rocking out with a worship band or preaching an hour-long sermon, for instance. But if we notice who is missing from these activities and ask why, we might be able to come up with some other, more inclusive, alternatives. And our fellowship will be richer because of it.

DEEPEN THE PAIN

Call me melancholy, but Advent and Lent are my favorite seasons in the church calendar. The dark purple. The sense of yearning for what has not yet come. The plaintive songs of waiting. The reminders of our sin, our impending death, and the present darkness. Not all Christian traditions observe these seasons, which is a loss. Not being able to bring our darker feelings to church cuts us off from our full humanity, as Taylor said. It flattens what would be joy into saccharine platitudes.

When I was in the worst of my pain, I felt most at home in church during Advent and Lent. I didn't feel forced to contort my face into a smile during worship. I could wear my true emotions—my confusion, my sadness—and find their resonance in the somber, brooding mood of the church. I finally felt I was not alone. It seemed normal to struggle and suffer. And that sense of being accompanied led to hope, to courage. Surrounded by the cries of the church—"Come, Lord Jesus" and "How long, O Lord?"—I was able to trust that my own cries would be heard. That I would make it through the tunnel to the other side.

Lament and hope go hand in hand, writes J. Todd Billings. We lament that things are not as they should be, that God's faithfulness is not apparent. But lament, Billings says, is "an expression of trust in his promises."[7] Lament opens the space for us to prepare—and truly hope—for God's kingdom to come in fullness. You might say that lament precedes hope.

Yet in many churches, lament has been largely evacuated from the sanctuary. We sing psalms of triumph and exultation, but shy away from the hard psalms, the ones that don't have a happy ending, like Psalm 88: "I am shut in so that I cannot escape; my eye grows dim through sorrow. . . . O LORD, why do you cast me off? Why do you hide your face from me?" (vv. 8-9, 14). The psalm ends with, "You have caused friend and neighbor to shun me; my companions are in darkness" (v. 18).

This psalm tells it like it is. It is true to our most wrenching human experiences. We are left hanging, waiting for resolution. Just like it is in life. And somehow, this is a comfort more than any triumphant song that glosses over the grief and tears that necessarily precede the victory. When we do not include expressions of lament like these in our corporate worship, it is no wonder that people drop away from church in the hard times. There is no place for them to bring their difficult emotions to God. No place for them to be honest.

Seasons like Advent and Lent, and their accompanying songs of lament, offer such a place. We can build these seasons of corporate grief work into all our church communities. We can also sit at the feet of marginalized communities who have long histories of injustice and suffering.

Grace, who has lived with chronic migraines since she was three, has mourned for the things pain has taken away from her. As a college student, she has lost opportunities for relationship, spending days when she would have been with peers on retreats or at trainings instead curled up in her bed in the dark. Once, she planned a "Friendsgiving" and started having a migraine as they prepared the meal. She spent the rest of the time upstairs, listening to her friends finish cooking and enjoy the meal she had planned.

Learning to grieve losses is part of Grace's spiritual growth these days. Specifically, she's learned from the African American community (she's white). "There's a role and a place and a discipline to it—the idea of crying out to God. There's space for frustration and anger and verbalizing these things publicly and privately," she said. Grace has benefited from being in spaces where lament is affirmed and practiced regularly. Her pain from migraines may be different from her friend's pain that comes from reckoning with what it means to be black in America. Grace sometimes feels like hers is nothing by comparison, not even worth mentioning. But keeping her pain to herself isolates her, while verbalizing it (with wisdom and discretion) brings her in. By sharing in others' sufferings and allowing others to share hers, Grace understands now that their unique experiences of loss "are all threaded together."

That is what spaces of lament can do. They take the individual experience of pain to a deeper level. They say, "This is what it means to be human. We are all in this together." Henri

Nouwen writes that this is the call of all who follow in the ministry of Jesus—to deepen the pain:

> When people come with their loneliness to ministers, they can only expect that their loneliness will be understood and felt, so that they no longer have to run away from it but can accept it as an expression of the basic human condition. When a woman suffers the loss of her child, ministers are not called upon to comfort her by telling her that she still has two beautiful healthy children at home; they are challenged to help her realize that the death of her child reveals her own mortal condition, the same human condition that the minister and others share with her. . . . Therefore ministry is a very confrontational service. It does not allow people to live with illusions of immortality and wholeness. It keeps reminding others that they are mortal and broken, but also that with the recognition of this condition, liberation starts.[8]

The church does have a role in seeking to relieve pain and suffering. This is part of our call to love our neighbors and affirm life. Yet there is only so much we can do on this side of the resurrection. In the meantime, while we walk "in the valley of the shadow of death," the ministry of relieving pain must be coupled with the ministry of deepening pain. We bring the pain down to a shared level. And somehow, in the depths, the burden is lighter.

THE MINISTRY OF THE BROKEN

If one of the callings of the church is to deepen the pain, those who have undergone the most suffering may be the most equipped to minister. They know what it feels like at the edge of life.⁹ They have been through our worst fears. Suffering has pried their fingers off the driver's wheel of life, and now, sitting in the passenger's seat, they notice the landscape. They are guides who point out landmarks we would miss. They tell us, "It seems you are going in circles in a forest, passing by the same trees over and over. But from God's perspective, you're on the straightest path from point A to point B. You are not lost. Others have traveled here."

This is what my friend Barbara told me when I met with her regularly to pray during the worst of my chronic pain. Barbara had her own share of pain. She had been bedridden for weeks with back issues. I remember staring at her lace-up white sneakers as I poured out a stream of woes and tears, and then looking up at her face, wondering what reaction she might have to my "heresies." She never seemed surprised.

When I told Barbara I didn't want to get any closer to God if *this* was what it was like for those who sought his face, she sat with me in my fear and anger. Then she told me God's love is like an ocean: When you first put your feet in, it's fun and exhilarating. But then, you get farther out, and the waves are really violent. Sometimes they just about knock you over and drown you. It makes you want to get back on dry land. But then, when you get even farther out, the waves get still. In the middle of the ocean, the water gently lulls you, and you float without needing your feet to touch the ground. It's no longer turbulent. You become one with the ocean.

Barbara put my darkness on a spiritual map. Though it felt as if I had fallen off the map, and that my experiences were marginal to the life of faith, she reassured me that they were, in actuality, well within the range of normal. She pointed me to saints like Thérèse of Lisieux and John of the Cross, who went through their own dark nights of the soul. Barbara deepened the pain. She gave me the courage to keep moving forward.

Listening, naming, and deepening the pain—these are all gifts that people with chronic illness (and all who know suffering well) can offer. "When you are broken and wounded, you can be with broken and wounded people in whole new ways. You're not afraid of it anymore," said Pat. How can we as the church move broken people from the periphery, where they are *ministered to* (prayed for by ministers in the side aisles, seated in the places reserved for the handicapped), to the center, where they *are the minsters*, offering their brokenness as a point of connection and a source of healing?

There are times, when we are groping along in the dark night of the soul, that we feel we have nothing to give that would benefit others. Our eyes are "dim through sorrow," as the psalmist says (Psalm 88:9). Our faith legs are shaky, and we may need others to hold us up. For some, the dark night can last for years, even decades. We may never recover from our illness. The pain drags on, or even intensifies. Must we "get better" in order to move out of the margins and toward the center? Are positions of leadership and visible ministry only for those whose faith is sure, whose lives are "successful"—in other words, contain a job, a house, a spouse, and kids?

Theologian Frederick Niedner holds up the life of Mother Teresa as an example of fruitful ministry in times of darkness. After her death, it was discovered that this saint of a woman, who devoted her life to caring for the dying on the streets of Calcutta, lived through extended periods of darkness and loneliness, perhaps for the entire second half of her life. The woman whom many uphold as a paragon of faith wrote, "The place of God in my soul is blank."[10] And yet Mother Teresa continued to offer succor to those on the edge of life. She gave skin to God's love and provision. "The truest blessing we find and the only faithfulness we exercise in times of clawing emptiness may well come not in being able to see an answer to our prayers," Niedner writes, "but in finding ourselves the embodiments of God's merciful response to another's prayers for mercy."[11]

So, no. We don't have to "get better" in order to minister. But we might have to take down some of our conceptual frameworks around ministry.

There are some basic programmatic elements that make it hard for people with chronic illnesses or other disabilities to serve in the church. Many ministry positions require long-term commitments or being on your feet for extended periods—teaching Sunday school or serving at a food pantry, for instance. People with chronic illnesses often cannot predict their pain or fatigue levels from day to day. They might be able to attend part of an event but need to go home in the middle or attend one week but not the next. The assumption that a faithful servant of the Lord will be at the church whenever the doors are open leaves many chronically ill people with a sense of being less than faithful.

Instead of sending the message that ministry is obligatory, churches can communicate that ministry is a gift—both for the giver and the receiver. We serve out of joy, because we have something we want to give. The rest of the church receives that service with gratitude, without expecting the same or more each time. Having an attitude of flexibility and open receptivity allows people to serve when they can without pressure to be constantly serving—and burning themselves out.

The ability to name limits—"this is what I can do and this is what I can't"—is also a gift to the church. Pat could serve at her church's coffee hour, but she needed help getting the boxes of supplies out of the closet. She shared that information, and now some younger men help her. "It enriches everybody's lives. They know that they're helping me, they know I appreciate it, and I don't have to fake it," she said. Pat modeled having healthy limits, thereby leading others toward wholeness.

UPSIDE-DOWN KINGDOM

The gifts we bring to church are not necessarily what we "give."

Again, Joyce Ann Mercer's theology on the vocation of older adults is helpful here. As we looked at in chapter six, she suggests that older adults' calling comes out of what they *call out* in others—care, attentiveness, patience, slowing down. These are all "practices, habits, and dispositions of faithful people,"[12] ones we are called to exercise in the presence of anyone who is vulnerable, sick, very old, very young, or simply different.

When people can't "give" in the ways we expect, it's an opportunity, an invitation from God to pay attention to the other surprising gifts we might receive. Disability advocate Judith Snow tells the story of Miriam, a woman with intellectual disabilities who lived in the same co-op with her for a season. Miriam regularly walked into others' apartments and asked awkward questions. Nobody appreciated this, but because of Miriam they discovered they were all getting sick from the building's air ventilation system and then mobilized to get the building managers to fix it. Miriam had the gift of networking—connecting people who wouldn't otherwise be connected. The gifts we receive aren't always pleasant though, Snow points out.

She details other gifts that communities receive in the presence of people with disabilities. For example, they are more ready to receive strangers and extend hospitality.

Teachers get better at teaching—not just to those with disabilities but to everyone. Communities are more peaceful; they fight less because they have learned to value difference. They are also more grounded; since people with disabilities often take longer to do daily activities like walking to the car or eating, others are made to slow down with them, and are brought into the moment.[13]

I am reminded of Jesus' words, "Let the little children come to me, and do not stop them; for it is to such as these that the kingdom of heaven belongs" (Matthew 19:14). If we take his words to heart, we understand ourselves to be part of a kingdom where the poor, mourning, meek, hungry, thirsty, and persecuted are at the center (Matthew 5). We who are the movers and shakers of this world—the job holders, the bill payers, the lawmakers, and law enforcers—may see ourselves holding this place, but in God's economy, what you *do* is not nearly as important as who you *are*.

Little children know this inherently. That is why Jesus welcomes them to lead the procession, sticky hands, muddy feet, and all. As we get older and are deformed by the ways of this world, we must learn again what we knew as babes. Some of us come to these lessons through much suffering—illness, job loss, and the like. We become that which we once despised—unproductive, unable, incompetent. If we pay attention, though, we will find blessings here. Jesus says we will receive mercy. We will be comforted. We will see God.

Pat has learned to pay attention. One Sunday after Thanksgiving, she was having problems with her knee, to the extent that she was using a cane and could barely move. Nevertheless, she asked her friend Jane, who was homeless, if she could take her out to lunch. Jane declined, claiming she didn't want to be beholden to Pat. "But," Jane said, "I want you to come to lunch with me." At this point, Pat could have thought, *No, this is too weird. What am I getting myself into?* But she instead said, "Okay, Lord, let's go. I'm willing to see what this looks like." I'll let Pat finish the story:

> We got in the car, drove up the hill, basically, to another church that was having a Thanksgiving potluck. We got there before the service ended. I literally barely made it to the last row. I was just in agony. There was no way I could get up and go up front to Communion. The pastor saw me and came back and gave it to me.
>
> Then we get over to the table and sit down. I can't stand up to get a plate. I can't stand up at all and I'm using the cane, so I can't hold a cane and serve myself. Jane gets me a plate, comes and sits down, and these are all her friends. This is a person who is homeless, and I'm usually seeing myself as the one that's giving. Now I'm in her context and she's the hostess. She's introducing me to her friends. They don't know anything about me except I'm Jane's friend.
>
> It was such a fascinating turning-upside-down of things. She'd figured out a way for us to be together where I wasn't paying for it. She figured out a context, a place that was really comfortable for her, with people that she cared about, who liked her. It was just marvelous.

Pat continued, "I was totally helpless that particular day, just beyond able to do anything. It took me into a whole other world I never would have encountered. I met people I never would have met. Jane was able to give me this experience of being her guest that was . . ." She paused here for a moment, then picked up: "Jesus talked about banqueting tables. That was a banqueting experience. Totally opposite of any that I've ever experienced before."

THE JOURNEY CONTINUES

There is just the one body—
nothing is unrelated to the whole.

Li-Young Lee

"So, what happened?" my friend Caris asks me over coffee (tea for me). We are meeting so she can give me feedback on the first half of this book. What she means is, "Did you get better? How?"

I struggled with whether to include the details of how my years of chronic pain played out—the "resolution," so to speak. This is not a self-help book, an "I did this and I got better!" kind of book. Yet, I did get better. Some of it, I think, was time. Some of it was persisting to find health care practitioners who truly partnered with me in problem-solving. Some of it was self-care —attending to the needs of my body in simple things like eating nourishing food or doing yoga, which helped me to feel at ease again in a body that I felt had betrayed me.

Some of it is just a mystery. After about three years of constant pain, of always limping to walk, I got pregnant with our first child. During that nine months, something shifted in my joints, and by the end of my pregnancy, I was able to walk without pain and limping. I can't explain it.

That is not to say that my body went "back to normal." There is no normal, as I've come to realize. There is only this beautiful, well-used, well-loved, often-achy body, here and now. There are some spots along my left side that I've accepted will always be prone to aches in times of stress and overuse. When the pain flares up, as it has just in this past month, I take it as a reminder to slow down and be the human that I am. To rest, to do nothing, to take a hot shower, to get a massage. You don't need pain to have permission to do that. Yet sometimes it takes pain or some other setback to learn to do that.

I am still on the healing journey. I'm still learning to come home to my body. I live with the possibility that at any time the pain could return full force or even worse than before. Every day presents a stream of "triggers" that force me to choose—will I react in fear, resistance, and self-protection or will I breathe, stay present, and reach out?

The latest trigger is the COVID-19 pandemic. The virus has spread across countries and communities affecting people of all social statuses, but especially the poor and marginalized. We can only contain its spread if we understand that survival depends on action as a community, not just at an individual level. Our health depends on the preventative measures of others and on leaders to act wisely. We are not isolated home-steads when it comes to our health (though it may feel as if we are with social distancing). We are part of a whole.

I write this during a shelter-in-place order for the state of Illinois. The death toll in the United States is in the thousands. This pandemic is unprecedented in our recent collective memory.

Every morning, I wake up and the reality of our new normal washes over me. *Oh yeah, this. Living in the twilight zone still.*

But when I lean in, pushing past my initial feelings of anxiety, dread, and paralysis, I realize that maybe this experience is not so new. Yes, the pandemic is unprecedented in its global scale. But it reveals what we already know about our human condition. Our bodies are porous to the dangerous outside world. We can die from something invisible to the naked eye, from microscopic little balls of virus with spikes coming out like a crown. The threat lies within our borders, on our skin, in our lungs. Our bodies are so vulnerable.

Our lives hang by delicate gossamer threads woven into a web of reciprocal human actions. When we don't reach out to rethread the ties, to patch the holes in our communal lives, people will fall through the holes. Some will die. Sometimes breathing is hard, and you need others—people who make ventilators, people who fund and allocate and know how to run ventilators—to help you breathe. *Breathe in:* You are human. You could get COVID-19. *Breathe out:* You are not alone. We are all in this together.

The movements that I have learned on my journey with chronic pain are the same movements that can ground us in this era of coronavirus, or at any point when fear triggers that knee-jerk reaction to flee from our bodies. We move from being passive onlookers to active participants—partnering with God and members of our community to bring healing. We move from wishing ourselves back to a previous normal, to the way things were pre-pandemic, to accepting what is imperfect and noticing what is good about now. Now is the only moment we have. We move from seeing ourselves as free-floating agents protecting ourselves and our own to seeing ourselves as part of a wide, rich human community. We have the tools we need to recover. We just need to share with each other. We can move from fight, flight, or freeze reactions to presence, to reassociation. We are safer when we work together.

Unmoored by images of people in hospitals with tubes and cords sticking out and dire predictions about the economy, I drop anchor into my own skin. I come home. It is still a dangerous, uncertain place to be. What is that tickle in the back of my throat? Did I wash my hands after I handled that Amazon package? I breathe, and I look around me.

Here is my husband, sitting across from me at our dining table. I have poured some of my mom's homemade muscadine wine into two glasses, cut up some deep orange cheese in a bowl, and set out some bars of single-origin chocolate. (When others hoard toilet paper, I hoard highbrow chocolate.) We take turns unwrapping each bar from its gold foil and breaking off small squares. I put a piece from Maya Mountain, Belize, into my mouth, letting the chocolate melt over my tongue, trying to tease out the distinct flavors. "Butterscotch," Matt says. "Mmm, caramel," I reply. We look at the label, where the makers have printed what they taste: "Honey, sweet strawberry wine, chocolate ice cream." "Close, we got the creamy part right!" we laugh. On every bar, the makers say they taste something chocolate-related—chocolate cake, fudge, chocolate milk. Isn't that just saying that chocolate tastes like chocolate? We move on to the next bar.

By the time we're done, my breathing has slowed. I no longer feel that tightness in my chest. I'm present. I'm right here, right now. Here, there is grace. There is God. I am accompanied. I'm still hurting for all those people dying in hospital isolation. I'm still worried about my family, my neighbors, and the country.

My own body is still achy, imperfect. Yet I'm whole. I've tapped into a deeper source and reconciled my body and spirit. I'm moving forward now from a grounded place. A place of noticing, breathing, and waiting for something new to emerge.

I inhale. Lord Jesus Christ, have mercy on us. I exhale. Lord Jesus Christ, make us whole.

ACKNOWLEDGMENTS

*T*hough I am listed as the author, sometimes I feel like "mosaic-maker" would be a better way to describe my work. Like the mosaics that we and God make together out of the broken pieces of our lives, I have pieced together the stories, wisdom, and encouragement I have received from many people, some of whom I know personally and some of whom I know from afar. Directly or indirectly, many have contributed to this book. Those named below are by no means the only ones.

I'm grateful to the people who so graciously entrusted their stories of pain and illness to me, allowing me to weave them into my book. And I'm grateful to those who accompanied me in the depths of my pain and depression, who were not afraid to listen to my raw cries of confusion, including Melanie McKinney, Barbara Gauthier, and Katie Lindsey Nezat.

Beth Felker Jones, Cherith Fee Nordling, Kari Rauh, Angela Yarian, and others dialogued with me around the themes of my book in the early stages. The Her.manas showed me what is possible in the publishing world for a Christian woman with something to say. I'm especially grateful to Michelle Van Loon and Marlena Graves for their encouragement. Katelyn Beaty published my first freelance piece, "Asking Why to Chronic Pain at Age 22," and was the initial acquiring editor for this book. Thank you, Katelyn, for noticing and elevating my voice.

Many read parts of this book and provided feedback, including Caris Wood, Erin MacKinney, Emily Ramler, two anonymous outside readers, and the Writers of Norwich—Catherine McNiel, Aubrey Sampson, Kimberly Pelletier, and Laura Finch. Thank you each for your perspective.

Thank you to my editor, Al Hsu, for his seasoned guidance; to Helen Lee, who gave me a ride to the Festival of Faith and Writing once and heard my first timid book pitch; to Lori Neff; and to the other staff at InterVarsity Press who have worked to bring this book out into the world.

Catherine Penney, thank you for cheering me on and for commiserating on writing and mothering with me. Erika Olsen, thank you for checking in regularly and for speaking my love language of food and plants.

Some very wonderful people took care of my children so I could have the time to write this book, including the staff at the Treehouse, Jessie and Catherine Bass, Jennifer and Allison Manspeaker, and my mother, Yimin He. Speaking of my children, they have provided writing material, brought me out of my head and into my body, and surprised me with their support. My six-year-old, especially, was delighted to hear I had finished the book, gave me the most satisfying hug, and says that when he grows up he wants to make books, too, but he also wants to draw the pictures.

There is nothing I can say to fully express how grateful I am to my husband, Matt. He read multiple iterations of this book and gave up downtime on evenings and weekends so I could write. When I worried in our early years together that he would feel that my pain wasn't what he had signed up for, he told me he has never once regretted marrying me. Many of the thoughts I share in the book fermented and matured through conversations and long silences with this man.

All of you in my community show me who I am and who God is. Thank you.

NOTES

1 A JOURNEY BEGINS

[1]I say "most of us" because there are those who do not have the luxury of ignoring their bodies, even from the outset. People born with disabilities face from their very early days of life the reality of their bodies against what is "normal functioning." They must reckon earlier than most with what all of us will face at some point in our lives—our embodied limits and vulnerabilities.

[2]Elaine Scarry, *The Body in Pain* (Oxford: Oxford University Press, 1985), 35.

[3]Quoted in Parker Palmer, *A Hidden Wholeness* (San Francisco: Jossey-Bass, 2004), 3.

[4]Marva Dawn, *Being Well When We're Ill: Wholeness and Hope in Spite of Infirmity* (Minneapolis: Augsburg Books, 2008), 237.

[5]N. T. Wright, *Evil and the Justice of God* (Downers Grove, IL: InterVarsity Press, 2006), 116.

[6]Rates for chronic illness vary depending on what illnesses are counted as chronic. According to the Partnership to Fight Chronic Disease, 45 percent of American adults have some form of chronic illness, with that number projected to rise to nearly half (49 percent) by 2025. "The Growing Crisis of Chronic Disease in the United States," Fight Chronic Disease, accessed October 16, 2019, www.fightchronicdisease.org/sites /default/files/docs/GrowingCrisisofChronicDiseaseintheUSfactsheet _81009.pdf. The Centers for Disease Control and Prevention estimate that six in ten Americans have some form of chronic illness (cancer is included). "Chronic Diseases in America," Centers for Disease Control and Prevention, accessed March 15, 2020, www.cdc.gov/chronicdisease /resources/infographic/chronic-diseases.htm.

[7]I am deeply indebted to theologians within the disability community for opening the door to new ways to think about my body. You'll find some references in this book to works within the field of disabilities studies. I've only lightly waded into this field, but here are a few places to start if you're interested in exploring this area: Nancy Eiesland, *The Disabled*

God: Toward a Liberatory Theology of Disability (Nashville: Abingdon Press, 1994); Deborah Beth Creamer, *Disability and Christian Theology: Embodied Limits and Constructive Possibilities* (New York: Oxford University Press, 2008); Devan Stahl, ed., *Imaging and Imagining Illness: Becoming Whole in a Broken Body* (Eugene, OR: Cascade Books, 2018); and Shane Clifton, *Crippled Grace: Disability, Virtue Ethics, and the Good Life* (Waco, TX: Baylor University Press, 2018). My friend Bethany McKinney Fox, who also writes on disability—see *Disability and the Way of Jesus: Holistic Healing in the Gospels* (Downers Grove, IL: InterVarsity Press, 2019)—helped me compile this list.

[8]I recommend Kathryn Greene-McCreight's book *Darkness Is My Only Companion: A Christian Response to Mental Illness* (Grand Rapids, MI: Brazos Press, 2006) as a helpful starting point for thinking theologically about mental illness.

2 SPLIT AT THE CORE

[1]Plato, *Republic*, trans. and ed. Raymond Larson (Arlington Heights, IL: AHM Publishing Corporation, 1979), 174-80.

[2]Tara Owens, *Embracing the Body: Finding God in Our Flesh and Bone* (Downers Grove, IL: InterVarsity Press, 2015), 44.

[3]Jean Danielou, *From Glory to Glory: Texts from Gregory of Nyssa's Mystical Writings*, trans. and ed. Herbert Musurillo (Crestwood, NY: St. Vladimir's Seminary Press, 1998), 11-13.

[4]Ryan Bebej, interview with the author, February 25, 2019.

[5]Rebecca Randall, "Why Zika, and Other Viruses, Don't Disprove God's Goodness," *Christianity Today,* August 14, 2018, www.christianitytoday.com /ct/2018/august-web-only/why-zika-and-other-viruses-dont-disprove -gods-goodness.html.

[6]Robert Gnuse, *Misunderstood Stories: Theological Commentary on Genesis 1–11* (Eugene, OR: Cascade Books, 2014), 118-30; and Richard Middleton, "Death, Immortality, and the Curse: Interpreting Genesis 2–3 in the Context of the Biblical Worldview" (prepared for the Dabar Conference in Deerfield, Illinois on June 13-16, 2018). Middleton, for instance, argues that mortality is part of humanity's created state, not a curse resulting from the Fall. Among other evidence, he cites John Calvin, who, commenting on "you are dust, and to dust you shall return" (Genesis 3:19), notes that "what God declares belongs to man's *nature*, not his *crime* or *fault.*"

[7]Middleton, "Death, Immortality, and the Curse."

[8]Terence Fretheim, *Creation Untamed: The Bible, God, and Natural Disasters* (Grand Rapids, MI: Baker Academic, 2010), 13-15.

[9]Kat Eschner, "Those Little Birds on the Backs of Rhinos Actually Drink Blood," *Smithsonian Magazine*, September 22, 2017, www.smithsonianmag.com/smart-news/those-little-birds-backs-rhinos-actually-drink-blood-180964912/.

[10]Fretheim, *Creation Untamed*, 3.

[11]Sabrina Strings, "It's Not Obesity. It's Slavery: We know why Covid-19 is killing so many black people," *The New York Times*, May 25, 2020, www.nytimes.com/2020/05/25/opinion/coronavirus-race-obesity.html.

[12]R. Marie Griffith, *Born Again Bodies: Flesh and Spirit in American Christianity* (Berkeley: University of California Press, 2004), 24.

[13]Griffith, *Born Again Bodies*, 162-63.

[14]There has been an unfortunate and inaccurate conflation of thinness with health and fatness with illness. But not all whose bodies weigh more than the range of "normal" are unhealthy.

[15]Griffith, *Born Again Bodies*, 7.

[16]Max Weber, in his sociology classic, *The Protestant Ethic and the Spirit of Capitalism* (New York: Dover, 2003), argues that this anxiety was part of what made the never-ending growth logic of capitalism work. Protestants, in the shadow of not knowing whether they were part of the predetermined "elect," were always trying to produce more and work harder because these were outward signs of faith and salvation.

[17]Stephanie Paulsell, *Honoring the Body: Meditations on a Christian Practice* (San Francisco: Jossey-Bass, 2002), 18-19.

[18]For many with chronic conditions, looking beyond the local church to support groups online or in person can be a helpful way to find resources and support. On the other hand, one of my interviewees told me the support groups she tried weren't very helpful because people were in different places and some were "stuck."

[19]Tish Harrison Warren, "My Lord and Migraine," *The Well* (blog), January 14, 2016, https://thewell.intervarsity.org/blog/my-lord-and-migraine.

[20]Kate Bowler, *Everything Happens for a Reason and Other Lies I've Loved* (New York: Random House, 2018), xiv.

3 ELUSIVE HEALING

[1]Terence Fretheim, *Creation Untamed: The Bible, God, and Natural Disasters* (Grand Rapids, MI: Baker Academic, 2010), 13.

[2]Mario A. Russo, "Caring for Creation as New Creations," BioLogos, October 9, 2019, https://biologos.org/articles/caring-for-creation-as-new-creations.

[3]William J. Webb, *Slaves, Women and Homosexuals: Exploring the Hermeneutics of Cultural Analysis* (Downers Grove, IL: InterVarsity Press, 2001).

[4]Bromleigh McCleneghan, *Good Christian Sex: Why Chastity Isn't the Only Option—and Other Things the Bible Says About Sex* (San Francisco: HarperOne, 2016), 97.

[5]Brother Roger of Taizé, *The Sources of Taizé: No Greater Love* (Chicago: GIA Publications, 2000), 11.

[6]Joni Eareckson Tada, *A Place of Healing: Wrestling with the Mysteries of Suffering, Pain, and God's Sovereignty* (Colorado Springs: David C. Cook, 2010), 167.

[7]Nancy Eiesland, "Encountering the Disabled God," *PMLA* 120, no. 2 (March 2005): 584-86.

[8]Beth Felker Jones, *Marks of His Wounds: Gender Politics and Bodily Resurrection* (New York: Oxford University Press, 2007), 23.

[9]Krystine Batcho, "The Psychological Benefits—and Trappings—of Nostalgia," The Conversation, June 5, 2017, www.theconversation.com/the-psychological-benefits-and-trappings-of-nostalgia-77766.

[10]Liuan Huska, "Can Anti-Aging Treatments Offer Abundant Life?" *Christianity Today,* February 15, 2019, www.christianitytoday.com/ct/2019/march/can-anti-aging-treatments-offer-abundant-life.html.

[11]Bruce A. Carnes and S. Jay Olshansky, *The Quest for Immortality: Science at the Frontiers of Aging* (New York: W. W. Norton & Company, 2001).

[12]Many scholars document this ideal. For a good start, see R. Marie Griffith's book *Born Again Bodies: Flesh and Spirit in American Christianity* (Berkeley: University of California Press, 2004). Griffith traces in detail the cultural roots of these conceptions.

[13]Historically, Western medicine has been a predominantly white, male field, which affects the biases and values informing the field. Definitions of "normal" often take nonrepresentative segments of the population as the baseline. For instance, men have frequently been used as the default for clinical trials, which excludes the entire female population from the results. (See "When Does Medicine Leave Women Behind?," NPR, February 10, 2017, www.npr.org/2017/02/10/514153036/when-does-medicine-leave-women-behind; and JoAnna Klein, "Fighting the Gender Stereotypes that Warp Biomedical Research," *The New York Times,* May 30, 2019,

www.nytimes.com/2019/05/30/health/gender-stereotypes-research
.html. Another example: the earliest infant growth charts were based on
a sample of white, bottle-fed babies born in Yellow Springs, Ohio, between the 1920s and mid-1970s. (See Marlene Cimons, "Pediatric Growth
Charts Often Leave Parents Confused and Concerned," *Washington Post*,
June 11, 2012, www.washingtonpost.com/national/health-science/pediatric
-growth-charts-often-leave-parents-confused-and-concerned/2012/06
/08/gJQAadfgUV_story.html.)

[14]Ranjani Iyer Mohanty, "The Rise and Fall of Fat in India," *New York Times*,
September 14, 2011, www.nytimes.com/2011/09/15/opinion/15iht-edmo
hanty15.html.

[15]Joyce Ann Mercer, interview with the author, July 10, 2018.

[16]Antonio Regalado, "A Stealthy Harvard Startup Wants to Reverse Aging
in Dogs, and Humans Could Be Next," *MIT Technology Review*, May 9, 2018,
www.technologyreview.com/s/611018/a-stealthy-harvard-startup-wants
-to-reverse-aging-in-dogs-and-humans-could-be-next/.

[17]Yuval Noah Harari, *Homo Deus: A Brief History of Tomorrow* (New York:
HarperCollins, 2017), 353.

[18]For more on our recent attempts to reach for control and transcendence,
see Christina Bieber Lake's book *Prophets of the Posthuman: American
Fiction, Biotechnology, and the Ethics of Personhood* (Notre Dame, IN: University of Notre Dame, 2013).

[19]Kate Bowler, *Everything Happens for a Reason and Other Lies I've Loved*
(New York: Random House, 2018), 16.

[20]Bowler, *Everything Happens for a Reason*, 25-26.

[21]Peter Enns, *The Sin of Certainty: Why God Desires Our Trust More Than Our
"Correct" Beliefs* (New York: HarperCollins, 2016), 84-85.

[22]"Rick Aguilar Feels the Magnificence of Christ," CBN, accessed October
22, 2019, www1.cbn.com/video/rick-aguilar-feels-the-magnificence-of
-christ.

[23]J. Todd Billings, *Rejoicing in Lament: Wrestling with Incurable Cancer and
Life in Christ* (Grand Rapids, MI: Brazos Press, 2015), 115.

[24]Quoted in Billings, *Rejoicing in Lament*, 62-63.

[25]I'm sure I'm not the first person to interpret this story this way, though
I can't recall where I first heard it. My friend Erin MacKinney, though, was
the last person who discussed and deepened this idea with me.

[26]Sometimes—not always, and probably not even a majority of the time—
physical ailments can be manifestations of deep-seated trauma that has

not been dealt with fully. Psychiatrist Bessel van der Kolk writes, "After trauma, the world is experienced with a different nervous system. The survivor's energy now becomes focused on suppressing inner chaos, at the expense of spontaneous involvement in their life." However, the inner chaos still gets out, sometimes finding expression in a range of physical symptoms, including fibromyalgia, chronic fatigue, and other autoimmune diseases. *The Body Keeps the Score: Brain, Mind, and Body in the Healing of Trauma* (New York: Penguin Books, 2014), 53. Addressing trauma may not make the symptoms go away completely, but it may be part of the healing journey.

[27]I'm grateful to my friend Erika for articulating these phrases in telling me her own story of healing from anxiety.

4 THE MYTH OF MEDICAL MASTERY

[1]Thanks to Dara Horn, who, in her novel *Eternal Life* (New York: W. W. Norton & Company, 2018), likens the medical research laboratory to the Jewish altar of sacrifice, inspiring my own ruminations.

[2]"Life Expectancy in the United States," EveryCRSReport.com, March 3, 2005–August 16, 2006, www.everycrsreport.com/reports/RL32792.html.

[3]Aubrey de Grey, a longevity researcher running the SENS Research Foundation in California, has said that the first human to live to one thousand is already alive. Sofie Thorsen, "The First Human to Live to 1,000 Has Already Been Born," *Scenario Magazine*, September 15, 2017, www.scenariomagazine.com/the-first-human-to-live-to-1000-has-already-been-born.

[4]Rachel Naomi Remen, *Kitchen Table Wisdom: Stories That Heal* (New York: Riverhead Books, 1996), xxiii–xxiv.

[5]Remen, *Kitchen Table Wisdom*, 53.

[6]Remen, *Kitchen Table Wisdom*, 158.

[7]Quoted in Eula Biss, "Medicine and Its Metaphors," *Guernica*, September 2, 2014, www.guernicamag.com/medicine-and-its-metaphors.

[8]Atul Gawande, *Being Mortal: Medicine and What Matters in the End* (New York: Metropolitan Books, 2014), 70.

[9]Carol Burkhardt and Kathryn Anderson, "The Quality of Life Scale (QOLS): Reliability, Validity, and Utilization," *Health and Quality of Life Outcomes* 1, no. 60 (October 2003).

[10]Kelsey Fitzgerald, interview with the author, October 16, 2018.

[11]Among transhumanists, some argue that the vision of progress needs to be tempered by an ethic of love and compassion. See the work of Micah Redding, who calls himself a Christian transhumanist: www.micahredding .com.

[12]Christina Bieber Lake, *Prophets of the Posthuman: American Fiction, Biotechnology, and the Ethics of Personhood* (Notre Dame, IN: University of Notre Dame, 2013), xii-xiii.

[13]Lake, *Prophets of the Posthuman*, 192.

[14]I am borrowing these words from ethicist Devan Stahl, who writes, "Medical categories do not always capture my evolving understanding of my illness. I am not satisfied to grant medicine sole interpretation of my body. . . . Artists, philosophers, theologians, anthropologists, bioethicists, and many other scholars write out of rich traditions seeking to interpret the meaning of embodiment and illness." Devan Stahl, ed., *Imaging and Imagining Illness: Becoming Whole in a Broken Body* (Eugene, OR: Cascade Books, 2018), xxv.

[15]Marva Dawn, *Being Well When We're Ill: Wholeness and Hope in Spite of Infirmity* (Minneapolis: Augsburg Books, 2008), 207. Dawn discovered the term "stochastic art" from an article by Katrine Ierodiakonou and Jan P. Vandenbroucke in an issue of *The Lancet* published in 1993.

[16]Remen, *Kitchen Table Wisdom*, 224.

[17]Remen, *Kitchen Table Wisdom*, 228.

[18]Stanley Hauerwas, "Finite Care in a World of Infinite Need," *Christian Scholars Review* 38, no. 3 (Spring 2009): 327-33.

[19]John Swinton, foreword to Bethany McKinney Fox, *Disability and the Way of Jesus: Holistic Healing in the Gospels and the Church* (Downers Grove, IL: InterVarsity Press, 2019), x, italics original.

[20]I want to credit my friend Kimberly Pelletier for the idea that when we are present to our own needs, we are able to then be more present to others' needs.

[21]Bob Cutillo, *Pursuing Health in an Anxious Age* (Wheaton, IL: Crossway, 2016), 25-26.

[22]Eula Biss, *On Immunity: An Inoculation* (Minneapolis: Graywolf Press, 2014), 76.

5 THE BURDEN WOMEN BEAR

[1]DeLisa Fairweather and Noel R. Rose, "Women and Autoimmune Disease," *Emerging Infectious Diseases* 10, no. 11 (November 2004): 2005-11.

[2] Sarah Williams, "Why Women Report Being in Worse Health than Men," *Scientific American,* December 30, 2011, www.scientificamerican.com/article/why-women-report-being-in/.

[3] Diane Hoffman and Anita Tarzian, "The Girl Who Cried Pain: A Bias Against Women in the Treatment of Pain," *Journal of Law, Medicine, and Ethics* 28, no. 4 (March 2001): 13-27.

[4] Hoffman and Tarzian, "The Girl Who Cried Pain," 17, 19-21. The authors conduct an extensive literature review and this article summarizes multiple studies. See their references for the specific studies that demonstrate health care bias against women.

[5] Interestingly, in this study, female patients were viewed as experiencing more pain, anxiety, and disability than male patients (regardless of perceived attractiveness). This may be explained by women's tendency to be more expressive of their pain. Thomas Hadjistavropoulos, Bruce McMurty, and Kenneth Craig, "Beautiful Faces in Pain: Biases and Accuracy in the Perception of Pain," *Psychology and Health* 11, no. 3 (1996): 411-20.

[6] Emily Martin, "Pregnancy, Labor, and Body Image in the United States," *Social Science & Medicine* 19, no. 11 (1984): 1201-6.

[7] Rachel Jones, "PMS: The Monthly Fight with the Flesh," The Gospel Coalition, February 24, 2020, www.thegospelcoalition.org/article/fight-with-the-flesh/.

[8] Beth Felker Jones, *Marks of His Wounds: Gender Politics and Bodily Resurrection* (New York: Oxford University Press, 2007), 19.

[9] Jones, *Marks of His Wounds,* 19.

[10] Judith Butler, "Performative Acts and Gender Constitution: An Essay in Phenomenology and Feminist Theory," *Theatre Journal* 40, no. 4 (1988): 519-31.

[11] I have in mind some streams of evangelical Anglicanism in the United States. They have drawn heavily from Catholic teachings on the theology of the body. See Christopher West's work for examples.

[12] Beth Felker Jones's book *Marks of His Wounds* helped me in finding my way through the essentialist-constructivist landscape (see the first chapter) and imaging different theological possibilities (see the fourth and fifth chapters in particular).

[13] Jones, *Marks of His Wounds,* 14.

[14] "Pregnancy Mortality Surveillance System," Centers for Disease Control and Prevention, accessed February 17, 2019, www.cdc.gov/reproductivehealth/maternalinfanthealth/pregnancy-mortality-surveillance-system.htm.

[15]Nina Martin, "Black Mothers Keep Dying After Giving Birth. Shalon Irving's Story Explains Why," NPR, December 7, 2017, www.npr.org/2017/12/07 /568948782/black-mothers-keep-dying-after-giving-birth-shalon -irvings-story-explains-why.

[16]Nina Martin, "Black Mothers Keep Dying After Giving Birth."

[17]Arline Geronimus et al., "Do U.S. Black Women Experience Stress Related Biological Aging? A Novel Theory and First Population-Based Test of Black-White Differences in Telomere Length," *Human Nature* 21, no. 1 (2010): 19-38.

[18]Olivia Remes et al., "A Systematic Review of Reviews on the Prevalence of Anxiety Disorders in Adult Populations," *Brain and Behavior* 6, no. 7 (July 2016), https://onlinelibrary.wiley.com/doi/epdf/10.1002/brb3.497.

[19]Huan Song et al., "Association of Stress-related Disorders with Subsequent Autoimmune Disease," *JAMA* 319, no. 23 (2018): 2388-400.

[20]Kristin Wong, "There's a Stress Gap Between Men and Women: Here's Why It's Important," *New York Times*, November 14, 2018, www.nytimes .com/2018/11/14/smarter-living/stress-gap-women-men.html.

[21]Arlie Hochschild, *The Second Shift: Working Parents and the Revolution at Home* (New York: Penguin, 1989).

[22]Donna Haraway, *Simians, Cyborgs, and Women: The Reinvention of Nature* (New York: Routledge, 1991), 253.

[23]Adrienne Rich, *Essential Essays* (New York: W. W. Norton & Company, 2018), 99.

[24]Rich, *Essential Essays*, 99.

[25]Jeffrey Boyd, *Being Sick Well: Joyful Living Despite Chronic Illness* (Grand Rapids, MI: Baker Books, 2005), 24.

[26]Jacqueline Howard, "Around the World, Mothers Have Similar Response to Crying Baby, Study Finds," CNN, updated October 25, 2017, www.cnn .com/2017/10/23/health/moms-babies-crying-response-universal-study /index.html.

[27]Alison Stuebe, Karen Grewen, and Samantha Meltzer-Brody, "Association Between Maternal Mood and Oxytocin Response to Breastfeeding," *Journal of Women's Health* 22, no. 4 (2013): 352-61.

[28]Kate Hennessy, *Dorothy Day: The World Will Be Saved by Beauty* (New York: Scribner, 2017), 27-28.

[29]Christine D. Pohl, *Making Room: Recovering Hospitality as a Christian Tradition* (Grand Rapids, MI: Eerdmans, 1999), 191.

[30]"About L'Arche," L'Arche USA, accessed October 23, 2019, www.larcheusa .org/who-we-are.

[31]"In the same wound where the pangs of anxiety are seething, creative forces are also being born." Brother Roger of Taizé, *The Sources of Taizé: No Greater Love* (Chicago: GIA Publications, 2000), 11. This quote was first referenced in chapter three.

[32]Jones, *Marks of His Wounds*, 103.

[33]Lauren Winner, "Divine Contractions: God's Labor, Our Deliverance," *The Christian Century*, March 5, 2015, www.christiancentury.org/article /2015-02/divine-contractions.

[34]Vaishali Moulton, "Sex Hormones in Acquired Immunity and Autoimmune Disease," *Frontiers in Immunology* 9, no. 2279 (2018), www.ncbi.nlm .nih.gov/pmc/articles/PMC6180207.

[35]Kyle Sue, "The Science Behind 'Man-Flu,'" *BMJ* 359, no. 5560 (2017), www .bmj.com/content/359/bmj.j5560.full.

[36]Julie Morris, "A Story of Two Leaky Bodies," *The Christian Century*, January 10, 2017, www.christiancentury.org/article/first-person/story-two-leaky -bodies.

[37]Quoted in Morris, "A Story of Two Leaky Bodies."

[38]Matthew J. Milliner, "What Men Can Learn from Mary, Mother of Jesus," *New York Times*, March 25, 2020, www.nytimes.com/2020/03/25/opinion /annunciation-mary-jesus-men.html.

[39]Stephanie Paulsell, *Honoring the Body: Meditations on a Christian Practice* (San Francisco: Jossey Bass, 2002), 174.

6 VULNERABLE BODIES

[1]Ask me in person and I'll tell you the story behind the nickname.

[2]Thomas Reynolds, *Vulnerable Communion: A Theology of Disability and Hospitality* (Grand Rapids, MI: Brazos Press, 2008), 60.

[3]Ephraim Radner, interview with the author, June 27, 2018.

[4]Vanessa King, *10 Keys to Happier Living: A Practical Handbook for Happiness* (London: Headline Publishing Group, 2016), chapter 9.

[5]Sherry Turkle, *Reclaiming Conversation: The Power of Talk in a Digital Age* (New York: Penguin Books, 2015), 142.

[6]Turkle, *Reclaiming Conversation*, 143.

[7]Turkle, *Reclaiming Conversation*, 127.

[8]Turkle, *Reclaiming Conversation*, 131.

[9]Eula Biss, "Sentimental Medicine: Why We Still Fear Vaccines," *Harper's Magazine*, January 2013, www.harpers.org/archive/2013/01/sentimental -medicine.

¹⁰In *The Myth of the American Dream: Reflections on Affluence, Autonomy, Safety, and Power* (Downers Grove, IL: InterVarsity Press, 2020), D. L. Mayfield insightfully names and critiques some of the values underpinning this myth.

¹¹Lauren Winner, "Divine Contractions: God's Labor, Our Deliverance," *The Christian Century*, March 5, 2015, www.christiancentury.org/article/2015-02/divine-contractions.

¹²Winner, "Divine Contractions."

¹³Judith Snow, "It's About Grace!" March 22, 2016, www.youtube.com/watch?v=rl_vqXZJF0k.

¹⁴William C. Placher, *Narratives of a Vulnerable God: Christ, Theology, and Scripture* (Louisville, KY: Westminster John Knox, 1994), 70.

¹⁵Joyce Ann Mercer, "What Does Christian Vocation Look Like for the Elderly?," *The Christian Century*, June 23, 2017, www.christiancentury.org/article/features/what-does-christian-vocation-look-elderly.

¹⁶Joyce Ann Mercer, "Older Adulthood: Vocation at Life's End," in *Calling All Years Good: Christian Vocation Throughout Life's Seasons*, ed. Kathleen A. Cahalan and Bonnie J. Miller-McLemore (Grand Rapids, MI: Eerdmans, 2017), 178, 188.

¹⁷Mercer, "Older Adulthood," 184.

¹⁸Norman Wirzba, "Waking Up to the Anthropocene," *The Christian Century*, September 27, 2017, 27.

7 OUR HUMAN LIMITS

¹Deborah Beth Creamer, *Disability and Christian Theology: Embodied Limits and Constructive Possibilities* (New York: Oxford University Press, 2008).

²This paragraph is a paraphrase compiled from an interview with Cherith Nordling, "What Does It Mean to Be Human?," Grace Communion Seminary, accessed October 23, 2019, www.gcs.edu/mod/page/view.php?id=4423, and a personal interview, October 10, 2016.

³Marva Dawn, *Being Well When We're Ill: Wholeness and Hope in Spite of Infirmity* (Minneapolis: Augsburg Books, 2008), 230.

⁴For the science on how stress affects the body, including how it dampens the immune system, see Matt Richtel, *An Elegant Defense: The Extraordinary New Science of the Immune System* (New York: William Morrow, 2019), especially chapter 34.

⁵"The Growing Crisis of Chronic Disease in the United States," Fight Chronic Disease, accessed October 16, 2019, www.fightchronicdisease.org

/sites/default/files/docs/GrowingCrisisofChronicDiseaseintheUSfactsheet
_81009.pdf.

[6]Tessa Love, "Why Are Autoimmune Diseases on the Rise?" Elemental, April 10, 2019, https://elemental.medium.com/autoimmunity-is-a-disorder -of-our-time-a7f1c45d6907.

[7]Joni Eareckson Tada, *A Place of Healing: Wrestling with the Mysteries of Suffering, Pain, and God's Sovereignty* (Colorado Springs: David C. Cook, 2010).

[8]Wendell Berry, "The Real Work," *Standing by Words* (Berkeley, CA: Counterpoint, 1983), 97.

8 THE CRAFT OF SUFFERING

[1]Thank you to our backup doula (and, since then, placenta encapsulator) Deb Lawrence, for that birth handout and the helpful tips.

[2]Lee Ann Pomrenke, "3 Ways That Calling God 'Mother' Transforms Us," Sojourners, April 3, 2019, www.sojo.net/articles/3-ways-calling-god-mother -transforms-us.

[3]Parker Palmer, *A Hidden Wholeness* (San Francisco: Jossey-Bass, 2004), 178.

[4]Christina Bieber Lake, *Prophets of the Posthuman: American Fiction, Biotechnology, and the Ethics of Personhood* (Notre Dame, IN: University of Notre Dame, 2013), 11.

[5]Ephraim Radner, interview with the author, June 27, 2018.

[6]Vincent Joseph McNabb, *The Craft of Suffering: Verbatim Notes of Instructions on Suffering* (London: Burns, Oates, & Washbourne, 1936). The book is out of print now, but I found a copy for sale on Amazon for $125.86, if you are that interested.

[7]Thich Nhat Hanh, *No Mud, No Lotus: The Art of Transforming Suffering* (Berkeley, CA: Parallax Press, 2014).

[8]Sociologists Christian Smith and Melinda Lundquist Denton coined the term "moral therapeutic deism" in the book *Soul Searching: The Religious and Spiritual Lives of American Teenagers* (New York: Oxford University Press, 2005) to describe several commonly held beliefs among the teenagers they surveyed, including that religion is mainly concerned with feeling good and being happy and at peace with oneself.

[9]David Bentley Hart explores extensively the idea that the best news about the gospel is that suffering is in the end rendered meaningless, "intrinsically devoid of substance and purpose," in *The Doors of the Sea: Where Was God in the Tsunami?* (Grand Rapids, MI: Eerdmans, 2005), 35, 61.

[10]For an in-depth theology of Holy Saturday, see Shelly Rambo, *Spirit and Trauma: A Theology of Remaining* (Louisville, KY: Westminster John Knox, 2010), especially the chapter "Witnessing Holy Saturday."

[11]Corrie ten Boom, *The Hiding Place* (Grand Rapids, MI: Chosen Books, 2006), 227.

[12]Wendell Berry, *Hannah Coulter* (Berkeley, CA: Counterpoint, 2005), 58.

[13]Berry, *Hannah Coulter,* 70.

[14]Berry, *Hannah Coulter,* 58.

[15]For more on the stages of grief, see the classic by David Kessler and Elizabeth Kubler-Ross, *On Grief and Grieving: Finding the Meaning of Grief Through the Five Stages of Loss* (New York: Scribner, 2014).

[16]Ephraim Radner, *A Time to Keep: Theology, Mortality, and the Shape of a Human Life* (Waco, TX: Baylor University Press, 2016), 156.

[17]Stephanie Paulsell, *Honoring the Body: Meditations on a Christian Practice* (San Francisco: Jossey-Bass, 2002), 174-75.

[18]Beth Slevcove, *Broken Hallelujahs: Learning to Grieve the Big and Small Losses of Life* (Downers Groves, IL: InterVarsity Press, 2016), 64.

[19]Karen Kilby, "Suffering, Pain and Loss in Christian Theology," Research Seminars Series, University of Nottingham, December 18, 2012, Nottingham, UK, www.youtube.com/watch?v=jhp6vu8NL7Y.

9 A DIFFERENT WHOLENESS

[1]While chronic illness is traumatic, trauma can also lead to chronic illness. Bessel van der Kolk writes that after trauma, "the world is experienced with a different nervous system. The survivor's energy now becomes focused on suppressing inner chaos, at the expense of spontaneous involvement in their life." This can result in a range of physical symptoms—including fibromyalgia, chronic fatigue, and other autoimmune diseases. *The Body Keeps the Score: Brain, Mind, and Body in the Healing of Trauma* (New York: Penguin Books, 2014), 53.

[2]Van der Kolk, *The Body Keeps the Score,* 69.

[3]Emily Nagoski, *Come As You Are: The Surprising New Science That Will Transform Your Sex Life* (New York: Simon and Schuster, 2015), 118, 124-25.

[4]Van der Kolk, *The Body Keeps the Score,* 73.

[5]Van der Kolk, *The Body Keeps the Score,* 274.

[6]Nagoski, *Come As You Are,* 125.

[7]Nagoski, *Come As You Are,* 129.

[8]Van der Kolk, *The Body Keeps the Score,* 86.

[9]Van der Kolk, *The Body Keeps the Score,* 73.

[10]Shelly Rambo articulates a theology of remaining amidst trauma: "Perhaps the divine story is neither a tragic or triumphant one, but, in fact, a story of divine remaining, the story of love that survives." Shelly Rambo, *Spirit and Trauma: A Theology of Remaining* (Louisville, KY: Westminster John Knox, 2010), 172.

[11]Scott Cairns, *The End of Suffering: Finding Purpose in Pain* (Brewster, MA: Paraclete Press, 2009), 72-73.

[12]Cairns, *The End of Suffering,* 37-38.

[13]Tara Owens, *Embracing the Body: Finding God in Our Flesh and Bone* (Downers Grove, IL: InterVarsity Press, 2015), 231.

[14]Julian of Norwich, *Revelations of Divine Love*, Project Gutenberg ebook, September 2, 2016, www.gutenberg.org/files/52958/52958-h/52958-h.htm.

[15]Deborah Beth Creamer, *Disability and Christian Theology: Embodied Limits and Constructive Possibilities* (New York: Oxford University Press, 2008), 3.

[16]Parker Palmer, *A Hidden Wholeness* (San Francisco: Jossey-Bass, 2004), 3-4. Palmer is referencing Douglas Wood's meditation on a jack pine.

[17]Stephanie Paulsell, *Honoring the Body: Meditations on a Christian Practice* (San Francisco: Jossey-Bass, 2002), 18.

[18]Thich Nhat Hanh, *No Mud, No Lotus: The Art of Transforming Suffering* (Berkeley, CA: Parallax Press, 2014), 24.

[19]Van der Kolk, *The Body Keeps the Score,* 266.

[20]Van der Kolk, *The Body Keeps the Score,* 69, 257-58.

[21]Ira Glass and Jaime Lowe, "Ten Sessions," August 23, 2019, in *This American Life,* podcast, www.thisamericanlife.org/682/ten-sessions.

[22]Van der Kolk, *The Body Keeps the Score,* 261.

[23]Van der Kolk, *The Body Keeps the Score,* 263.

[24]Van der Kolk, *The Body Keeps the Score,* 337.

[25]Liuan Huska, "'Pointless' Bones, 'Flawed' Birth Spacing, and 'Broken' Genes: Why Our Flaws Alone Can't Disprove God's Purpose," *Christianity Today,* March 28, 2019, www.christianitytoday.com/ct/2019/march-web -only/pointless-bones-flawed-birth-spacing-and-broken-genes.html.

[26]Manny Fernandez and Sarah Mervosh, "For Some in Texas, Imelda's Heavy Rains Feel Like Harvey 2.0," *New York Times,* September 19, 2019, www.nytimes.com/2019/09/19/us/imelda-hurricane-harvey.html.

[27]Ira Flatow, "The Future of Soil Under a Changing Climate," September 14, 2018, in *Science Friday,* produced by Alexa Lim, podcast, 12:04, www.science friday.com/segments/the-future-of-soil-under-a-changing-climate.

[28]Richard Middleton, "Death, Immortality, and the Curse: Interpreting Genesis 2–3 in the Context of the Biblical Worldview" (prepared for the Dabar Conference in Deerfield, Illinois on June 13-16, 2018).

10 A COMMUNITY OF WOUNDED HEALERS

[1]Barbara Brown Taylor, *Leaving Church: A Memoir of Faith* (San Francisco: HarperOne, 2006), 147-48.

[2]Kate Bowler, *Everything Happens for a Reason and Other Lies I've Loved* (New York: Random House, 2018), 112-13.

[3]Parker Palmer, *A Hidden Wholeness* (San Francisco: Jossey-Bass, 2004), 132.

[4]This is a term from Henri Nouwen's book by that name, *Wounded Healer: Ministry in Contemporary Society* (New York: Doubleday, 2010).

[5]Katherine Harmon, "How Important Is Physical Contact with Your Infant?," *Scientific American,* May 6, 2010, www.scientificamerican.com /article/infant-touch.

[6]Nouwen, *Wounded Healer,* 68.

[7]J. Todd Billings, *Rejoicing in Lament: Wrestling with Incurable Cancer and Life in Christ* (Grand Rapids, MI: Brazos Press, 2015), 43.

[8]Nouwen, *Wounded Healer,* 99.

[9]Rachel Naomi Remen, *Kitchen Table Wisdom: Stories That Heal* (New York: Riverhead Books, 1996). Remen uses the phrase "people on the edge of life" to refer to the people she works with who have cancer. In an interview with Krista Tippett, she said, "The repository of wisdom are the ill people in our culture." "The Difference Between Curing and Healing," updated November 22, 2018, in *On Being,* podcast, 51:58, www.onbeing .org/programs/rachel-naomi-remen-the-difference-between-fixing-and -healing-nov2018/.

[10]Quoted in Frederick Niedner, "How Does One Pray About Cancer?" *The Christian Century,* March 22, 2016, www.christiancentury.org/article/2016 -03/lord-have-mercy.

[11]Niedner, "How Does One Pray About Cancer?"

[12]Joyce Ann Mercer, "What Does Christian Vocation Look Like for the Elderly?," *The Christian Century,* June 23, 2017, www.christiancentury.org/article /features/what-does-christian-vocation-look-elderly.

[13]Judith Snow, "It's All About Grace!" March 22, 2016, www.youtube.com /watch?v=rl_vqXZJF0k.

ABOUT THE AUTHOR

*L*iuan Huska is a freelance writer who explores how the issues that affect us daily intersect with the deepest questions in our lives: Who are we? Where is God in all of this? How now shall we live? She has written on topics from immigration to sexuality in publications including *Christianity Today*, *The Christian Century*, Sojourners, Hyphen, and *Geez*. She brings an anthropologist's lens to her writing, having studied at Wheaton College in Wheaton, Illinois, and at the University of Chicago.

Liuan is 1.5 generation immigrant, born in China and raised in Southern California and parts of South and Southeast Texas. She and her husband, Matt, enjoy traveling with their three little boys, ages one, four, and seven. They live in West Chicago, Illinois. Connect with her through email at authorliuanhuska@gmail.com or on Twitter @LiuanHuska.

Bonus materials for *Hurting Yet Whole* are available at www.liuanhuska.com/resources.